THE

SOURCES OF HEALTH

AND

THE PREVENTION OF DISEASE;

OR,

MENTAL AND PHYSICAL HYGIENE.

BY

JOHN A. TARBELL, M.D.

MEMBER OF THE MASSACHUSETTS MEDICAL SOCIETY AND OF THE HOMŒOPATHIC NATIONAL INSTITUTE.

BOSTON:
OTIS CLAPP, 23, SCHOOL STREET.
NEW YORK: WM. RADDE.
1850.

BOSTON:
PRINTED BY JOHN WILSON,
No. 21, School-street.

CONTENTS.

CHAPTER.		PAGE.
I.	On Food	3
II.	On Drink	36
III.	On Air	64
IV.	On Exercise	80
V.	On Bathing	93
VI.	On Clothing	104
VII.	On Sleep	109
VIII.	On Occupations	114
IX.	On Drugs	122
X.	On Mental Causes of Disease	136
XI.	On Invisible Influences Affecting Health	144
XII.	On Homœopathy	152

PREFACE.

WHILE publications without number have issued from the press, inculcating various modes of alleviating the sufferings of the sick, — while opposing systems of practical medicine, based upon fallacious theories, count their editorial advocates by thousands, few comparatively have been the works treating of preventive measures best calculated to counteract the manifold causes which give rise to disease. A proper understanding of the nature of those causes, and of their action upon mental and physical health, will tend materially to lessen the chances of illness, and to improve the condition of all classes. The study of Anatomy, which has recently been, to some extent, introduced as a branch of elementary education, is of far less importance than the extension of knowledge respecting those influences, affecting human health, with which all are necessarily and continually brought into contact.

The object of the present work is to acquaint the reader with the character of those agents which exert an injurious influence upon health, and to afford instruction regarding means of adoption most practicable for the successful resistance of such evil agents. The views of Hahnemann in this particular will be in an especial manner regarded. No believer in his doctrine can be insensible to the importance of attending even to the minutiæ of matters modifying health and involving life.

The Author proffers claims to but little originality, and is far from presuming that the limited views herein offered do full justice to the important subject of Hygiene. But the laborers have been extremely few in such a vast field; and even this feeble attempt to aid in the removal of those physical obstructions which impede the development of man's spiritual nature would not have been made, but in the hope of inducing writers of more ability to pursue the like path.

THE SOURCES OF HEALTH.

THE most important of those morbific influences which constantly tend, especially in civilized life, to the deterioration of health, are Indigestible Food, Artificial Drinks, Vitiated Air, and Sedentary Habits. These several subjects will be treated of under their respective heads; and attention will be afterwards directed to the various agents which have a less immediate but still most influential bearing upon the physical well-being of mankind.

CHAPTER I.

ON FOOD.

A GENERAL description of the digestive and assimilative processes by which aliment becomes incorporated with the system for the support of life, although more strictly physiological than hygienic, will not be an inappropriate introduction to the subject under consideration.

The presence of food, which has been introduced into the mouth, stimulates, in connection with the mechanical act of mastication, certain salivary glands therein situated, and causes them to pour out an increased quantity of their peculiar secretion. This fluid, surrounding and penetrating the masticated mass, not only facilitates its passage down the canal (œsophagus) to the stomach, but assists in dissolving it. Having entered the stomach, another more powerful solvent (the gastric juice) mixes with the salivary secretion, and the food is subjected to their joint action, until it is converted into a soft paste, called "chyme." The warmth maintained in the stomach by the determination of blood to the vessels of that and the neighboring organs during this exercise, and the continual contraction of its muscular membrane upon that contained therein, also conduces to the formation of chyme. Then this softened material passes out of the portion of the stomach, opposite to that where it entered, into the intestine; where it is again acted upon by other secretions, and changed into a fluid state, denominated "chyle;" in which form the aliment, which has passed through the different stages of mastication, deglutition, chymification, and chylification, is absorbed by innumerable minute vessels, the mouths of which line the inner membrane of the intestinal tube that is continued from the stomach. The chyle is conveyed through these small vessels into the blood; and the latter is distributed, with its nutritious particles, to every portion of the frame, — thus ever engaged in repairing the losses which are ever occurring. The residue of the material, that which may have been undigested, or which cannot be converted into nourishment, passes down the canal, or rather through it, — since the intestine is so involuted as, in one portion, to have an upward direction, — and is thrown out of the system as useless.

Now, there exists a great difference in the nature of alimentary substances with regard to their conversion into that fluid which sustains life. Many, by their indigestible properties, cannot be transformed with facility into "chyme." Oily, tendinous, and cartilaginous food tax the powers of digestion more than fibrinous and glutinous substances. Some articles, such as skins of fruit, the stones, seeds, &c. which imprudent persons are often pleased to force down their throats, continue unaltered and of course unassimilated, ultimately rejected as foreign substances, or accumulating in the intestinal canal, to inflict uneasiness and distress, until removed by the violent action of deleterious purgatives. It is evident that every thing received into the stomach, which disturbs the powers of digestion, and does not contribute to the production of healthy chyle, must be more or less injurious. All crude, medicinal substances, independent of their positively poisonous qualities, interfere with salutary digestive action, and invariably derange the secretions. Yet one would suppose, from the avidity and frequency with which many would-be invalids swallow the nauseous preparations of the druggists, that they labored under the delusion that medicines were nutritious.

It must not be inferred, however, that every description of food not easily digestible, is, on that account, innutritious. On the contrary, a quantity of fat meat affords nearly four times as much nutriment as the same amount of lean meat, although the former is with much greater difficulty digested; in fact, undergoes but little, if any, alteration in the stomach. After it has moved thence, it must mix with the alkali of the bile, before it is in a fit state to impart nourishment.

In this connection, it may be proper to advert to the prevalent but entirely erroneous opinion, that *bile* is frequently present in large quantities in the stomach, and that its existence there is the cause of much indisposition. Bile is a secretion of the liver; and the duct conveying it from that organ, to act upon the chyme, enters the alimentary canal some inches below the lower orifice of the stomach. It there performs its object, passing down with the digested mass, which is propelled by a vermicular movement of the intestines, and cannot enter the stomach except by a strong inverted action. A portion may, it is true, be forced into the stomach in this manner, when some unconcocted substance therein is demanding all the activity of digestion. But, if there, it should be suffered to remain. The pernicious agency of emetics is not confined to the simple removal, by a most unnatural mode of exit, of that which is needed to facilitate digestion, perhaps in an emergency, but augments the supposed evil by stimulating the intestine to increased inverted action, thereby compelling a greater flow of bile into the stomach, when it is required elsewhere. Again, the absurd practice of endeavoring to remove an imagined accumulation of bile by purgatives, particularly by that most injurious of all substances which can enter the human system, viz. calomel, cannot be too strongly reprobated. It is the very extreme of folly to attempt the regulation of the bilious secretion by such medicines. They more frequently originate the very condition which they are expected to remove. The extent of positive mischief resulting from the use of "bilious pills," and other like preparations recommended by educated and uneducated empirics, is incalculable. When men will consent to the exercise of a reasonable degree of self-denial in the indulgence of appetite, and devote some little attention to the study of the laws of health, there will be reason to expect, even among the desperate advocates of Allœopathic doses, that the custom of such wholesale drugging will be abandoned.

An excellent opportunity of ascertaining the comparative digestibility of individual articles of food by actual observation, occurred in the year 1822. A young Canadian received by accident a gun-shot wound in the left side, which penetrated the stomach. The attending surgeon, Dr. Beaumont of the army, thus describes this remarkable case: —

"The charge, consisting of powder and duck-shot, was received in the left side, blowing off the integuments to the size of a man's hand, breaking some of the ribs, lacerating the lower portion of the left lung, and penetrating the stomach. On the fifth day, sloughing took place; portions of the lung, bones, and stomach separated, leaving an opening in the latter large enough to admit the whole length of the finger into its cavity; and also a passage into the chest half as large as his fist. After one year the wound closed, leaving the orifice into the stomach, which remained open two and a half inches in circumference. For some months the food could be retained only by wearing a compress; but finally a small fold of the villous coat of the stomach began to appear, which gradually increased till it filled the aperture, and acted as a valve, so as completely to prevent any efflux from within, but to admit of being easily pushed back by the finger from without."

Taking every advantage of the chance thus offered, which never happened before and may never happen again, of becoming intimately acquainted with the progress of digestion, Dr. Beaumont experimented perseveringly and unobstructedly for several months, and the following were the inferences drawn by him from minute and most accurate observation, viz.: —

1. That hunger is the effect of a *distension* of the vessels that secrete the gastric juice.

2. That the process of *mastication*, *insalivation*, and *deglutition*, in an abstract point of view, do not in any way affect the digestion of the food; or, in other words, when food is introduced directly into the stomach in a finely divided state, without these previous steps, it is as readily and as perfectly digested as when they have been taken.

3. That *saliva* does not possess the properties of an alimentary solvent.

4. That the *agent* of chymification is the gastric juice.

5. That the pure gastric juice is fluid, *clear and transparent;* without odor, a little salt, and perceptibly acid.

6. That it contains free muriatic acid, and some other active *chemical* principles.

7. That it is never found *free* in the gastric cavity, but is always excited to discharge itself by the introduction of *food* or other irritants.

8. That it is secreted from vessels distinct from the mucous follicles.

9. That it is seldom obtained pure, but is generally mixed with mucus and sometimes saliva. When pure, it is capable of being kept for months, and perhaps for years.

10. That it *coagulates* albumen, and afterward dissolves the *coagulum*.

11. That it *checks* the progress of putrefaction.

12. That it acts as a *solvent* of food, and alters its properties.

13. That, like other chemical agents, it *commences* its action on food as soon as it comes in contact with it.

14. That it is capable of combining with a certain and fixed *quantity* of food; and, when more aliment is presented for its action than it will dissolve, disturbance of the stomach or "indigestion" will ensue.

15. That its action is facilitated by the *warmth* and *motion* of the stomach.

16. That it becomes intimately *mixed* and *blended* with the ingestæ in the stomach by the motions of that organ.

17. That it is *invariably* the *same substance*, modified only by *admixture* with other fluids.

18. That the motions of the stomach produce a constant *churning* of its contents, and *admixture* of food and gastric juice.

19. That these motions are in two directions, *transversely* and *longitudinally*.

20. That *no other* fluid produces the same effect on food that gastric juice does, and that it is the only solvent of aliment.

21. That the action of the stomach and its fluids is the same on *all kinds* of diet.

22. That *solid* food, of a certain texture, is easier of digestion than fluid.

23. That *animal* and *farinaceous* aliments are more easy of digestion than *vegetable*.

24. That the susceptibility of digestion does not, however, depend altogether upon *natural* or *chemical* distinctions.

25. That digestion is facilitated by *minuteness of division* and *tenderness of fibre*, and retarded by opposite qualities.

26. That the *ultimate principles* of aliment are always the same, from whatever food they may be obtained.

27. That *chyme* is *homogeneous*, but variable in its *color* and *consistence*.

28. That, toward the latter stages of chymification, it becomes more *acid* and *stimulating*, and passes more rapidly from the stomach.

29. That the *inner coat* of the stomach is of a pale *pink* color, varying in its hues according to its full or empty state.

30. That, in health, it is sheathed with mucus.

31. That the appearance of the interior of the stomach *in disease* is essentially different from that of its *healthy* state.

32. That stimulating *condiments* are *injurious* to the healthy stomach.

33. That the use of *ardent spirits always* produces disease of the stomach, if persevered in.

34. That *water*, *ardent spirits*, and most other *fluids*, are not affected by the gastric juice, but pass from the stomach soon after they have been received.

35. That the *quantity* of food generally taken is more than the wants of the system require; and that such excess, if persevered in, generally produces, not only functional aberration, but disease of the coats of the stomach.

36. That *bulk* as well as *nutriment* is necessary to the articles of diet.

37. That *bile* is not ordinarily found in the stomach, and is *not* commonly *necessary* for the digestion of the food; but,

38. That, when *oily food* has been used, it assists its digestion.

39. That *oily food* is difficult of digestion, though it contains a large proportion of the nutrient principles.

40. That the *digestibility* of aliment does not depend upon the *quantity* of nutrient principles that it contains.

41. That the natural temperature of the stomach is about 100° Fahrenheit.

42. That the temperature is not elevated by the ingestion of food.

43. That *exercise* elevates the temperature; and that sleep or rest, in a recumbent position, depresses it.

44. That gentle exercise facilitates the digestion of food.

45. That the time required for that purpose is various, depending upon the quantity and quality of the food, state of the stomach, &c.; but that the time ordinarily required for the disposal of a moderate meal of the fibrous parts of meat, with bread, &c. is from three to three and a half hours.

The following results of Dr. Beaumont's experiments exhibit the time required for the digestion of different articles of food, prepared in the various ways of cooking usually adopted: —

			Hours.	Min.
Rice	Boiled	. Digested in .	1	
Pig's Feet, soused .	,,	. . . .	1	
Tripe, soused . . .	,,	. . . .	1	
Eggs, whipped . .	Raw	. . . .	1	30
Trout, Salmon, fresh	Boiled	. . . .	1	30
,, ,, ,,	Fried	. . . .	1	30
Apples, sweet . .	Raw	. . . .	1	30
Venison-steak . .	Broiled	. . . .	1	35
Brains	Boiled	. . . .	1	45
Sago	,,	. . . .	1	45
Tapioca	,,	. . . .	2	
Barley	,,	. . . .	2	
Milk	,,	. . . .	2	
Liver, beef's, fresh .	Broiled	. . . .	2	
Eggs, fresh . . .	Raw	. . . .	2	
Codfish, cured, dry .	Boiled	. . . .	2	
Apples, sour . . .	Raw	. . . .	2	
Cabbage, with vinegar	,,	. . . .	2	
Milk	,,	. . . .	2	15
Eggs, fresh . . .	Roasted	. . . .	2	15
Turkey, wild . . .	,,	. . . .	2	18
Turkey, domestic .	Boiled	. . . .	2	25
,, ,, .	Roasted	. . . .	2	30
Gelatine	Boiled	. . . .	2	30
Goose	Roasted	. . . .	2	30
Pig, sucking . . .	,,	. . . .	2	30
Lamb, fresh . . .	Broiled	. . . .	2	30
Beans, pod . . .	Boiled	. . . .	2	30
Cake, sponge . . .	Baked	. . . .	2	30
Parsnips	Boiled	. . . .	2	30

			Hours.	Min.
Potatoes, Irish . .	Roasted .	Digested in .	2	30
,, ,, . .	Baked	. . . .	2	30
Cabbage, head . .	Raw	. . . .	2	30
Spinal Marrow . .	Boiled	. . . .	2	40
Chicken	Fricassee	. . . . . .	2	45
Custard	Baked	. . . .	2	45
Beef	Boiled	. . . .	2	45
Oysters	Raw	. . . .	2	55
Eggs	Soft Boiled	. . . . . .	3	
Beef, fresh, lean, rare	Roasted	. . . .	3	
Beef-steak	Broiled	. . . .	3	
Pork, salted . . .	Raw	. . . .	3	
,, ,, . . .	Stewed	. . . .	3	
Mutton, fresh . .	Broiled	. . . .	3	
,, ,, . .	Boiled	. . . .	3	
Chicken Soup . .	,,	. . . .	3	
Dumpling, apple .	,,	. . . .	3	
Oysters	Roasted	. . . .	3	15
Pork-steak . . .	Broiled	. . . .	3	15
Pork, salted . . .	,,	. . . .	3	15
Mutton	Roasted	. . . .	3	15
Bread, corn . . .	Baked	. . . .	3	15
Carrot	Boiled	. . . .	3	15
Sausage	Broiled	. . . .	3	20
Flounder	Fried	. . . .	3	30
Oysters	Stewed	. . . .	3	30
Beef	Boiled	. . . .	3	30
Butter	Melted	. . . .	3	30
Cheese, old . . .	Raw	. . . .	3	30
Bread, wheaten, fresh	Baked	. . . .	3	30

			Hours.	Min.
Turnips	Boiled	. Digested in .	3	30
Potatoes, Irish . .	,,	. . . .	3	30
Eggs	Hard boiled	. . . . .	3	30
,, ...	Fried	. . . .	3	30
Green Corn & Beans	Boiled	. . . .	3	45
Beets	,,	. . . .	3	45
Salmon, salted . .	,,	. . . .	4	
Beef	Fried	. . . .	4	
Veal	Broiled	. . . .	4	
Fowls, domestic . .	Boiled	. . . .	4	
,, ,, . .	Roasted	. . . .	4	
Ducks, domestic . .	,,	. . . .	4	
Heart, animal . .	Fried	. . . .	4	
Beef, old, salted . .	Boiled	. . . .	4	15
Pork, salted . . .	Fried	. . . .	4	15
,, ,, . . .	Boiled	. . . .	4	30
Veal	Fried	. . . .	4	30
Ducks, wild . . .	Roasted	. . . .	4	30
Suet, mutton . . .	Boiled	. . . .	4	30
Cabbage, with vinegar	,,	. . . .	4	30
Suet, beef	,,	. . . .	5	3
Pork, fat and lean .	Roasted	. . . .	5	15

Here, then, we have facts clearly and irrefragably established, upon which to base reliable dietetic regulations. It will be observed that "minuteness of division" and "tenderness of fibre," according to the inferences drawn from Beaumont's trials, are necessary to the easy digestion of animal food; and that, in general, the latter contains more nutriment in a given bulk than vegetable food. Farinaceous preparations, as arrow-root, gruel, sago, &c. are quickly digested and assimilated, proving less stimulating than concentrated animal food, and hence better adapted for the system laboring under febrile action, or for inflammatory affections generally. All aromatic condiments are believed to be injurious, since they are more or less stimulating. The healthy stomach does not require artificial excitement to perform its work; and the same organ, when enfeebled, is rendered still more so by stimulants.

The regimen prescribed by the founder of the Homœopathic practice, long previous to the date of the above experiments, although drawn up with the view of excluding all food possessing any medicinal property that might counteract the operation of the remedies administered, will be found to have a close agreement with the facts here disclosed; and, though the system of diet is recommended with more direct reference to its consultation by invalids, yet it might be adhered to with decided profit by all. Old salted provisions, fat meats and oily substances, raw indigestible vegetables, highly seasoned food, and pastry, are especially forbidden during medical treatment; and the exclusion of such articles from the diet of every individual, in nearly all conditions and under nearly all circumstances, would undoubtedly tend to the prevention of disease.

In relation to the adaptation of certain kinds of

food to the requirements of the human system, modern researches in organic chemistry furnish interesting particulars as to the influence of temperature. According to Liebig, in respiration the lungs receive a greater quantity of oxygen in cold than in warm climates. A corresponding amount of carbon contained in food is required to unite with the oxygen, in order that a certain degree of animal heat should be kept up, and a proper balance between the loss and supply of materials preserved. Active exercise also, by accelerating respiration, augments the amount of air, and consequently of oxygen, which is inhaled. From food the system obtains carbon; and a portion of this carbon meets, through the medium of the lungs, with the oxygen supplied by the atmosphere, and a portion is thrown out in the form of carbonic acid. The carbon, together with a certain amount of hydrogen, constantly exhausted in this manner, must be as constantly replaced by equal quantities supplied in the food; and the amount of nourishment required for its support by the animal body must be in a direct ratio to the quantity of oxygen taken into the system. It is evident, therefore, that the aliment which is deficient in carbon will not be adequate for nourishment, under circumstances where an unusual amount of oxygen is inspired. For this reason, a diet containing but little carbon would not support the inhabitant of frozen regions, although it might suffice for the sustenance of the dweller in warm countries. Liebig remarks that "vital activity depends upon the mutual action of the elements of the food and the oxygen of the atmosphere combining together, and that the animal body acts, in this respect, as a furnace, which we supply with fuel. It signifies nothing what intermediate forms food may assume, what changes it may undergo in the body, the last change is uniformly the conversion of its carbon into carbonic acid, and of its hydrogen into water. In order to keep up in the furnace a constant temperature, we must vary the supply of fuel according to the supply of oxygen."

By reason of the excessive cold, and the consequent larger amount of oxygen afforded, the Greenlander lives upon train-oil, which contains nearly 80 per cent of carbon. Such food would very soon destroy the natives of warm or even temperate countries. The inhabitants of the torrid regions are nourished principally upon fruits which do not contain more than 12 per cent of carbon. But, while there is no doubt of the need of a proportionate supply of carbon for the oxygen received, there are other elements in food necessary for sustenance. It appears that wherever the human race is located, there food is furnished capable of nourishing the body and repairing its losses. That life may be supported by substances which are extremely difficult of digestion, and even by such as furnish a very minute proportion of nutriment according to their bulk, is certain; but that the standard of health must necessarily be low, under such conditions, is equally certain. A due amount of vital energy and consequent physical enjoyment depends upon the fulfilment of established laws, one of the most important of which relates to the quantity and quality of food.

The organization of the human digestive apparatus throughout, proves man to have been created omniverous, capable of subsisting upon animal and vegetable food, and acquiring the highest state of health upon a judicious combination of both. The proportion of each must vary according to the climate, the seasons, the occupation, and the age. For example, the inhabitants of northern climates require more animal food than those who live in warm latitudes. In the winter of temperate regions, more animal food is required than during summer. The laboring man needs more animal food than the sedentary. In manhood and in the decline of life, more is necessary than during the period previous to maturity.

ANIMAL FOOD,

As a general rule, is more quickly and easily digested than any other; but it is also more stimulating, and more productive of plethora, with all its evil consequences. If it predominates in the diet, while sufficient exercise is not taken, the system will be more liable to inflammatory diseases, and a foundation will also be laid for subsequent long-continued and obstinate disorders. It should constitute, in our climate, by much the smallest proportion of the quantity of food taken, and more especially by the inhabitants of a city.

The chief proximate principles of animal food are *fibrine*, *albumen*, *gelatine*, *oil*, and *caseine;* each of which will be briefly described.

Fibrine is found both in vegetables and animals. It constitutes the principal part of animal flesh, and enters largely into the composition of the blood. It is a solid, insoluble in water, becoming semi-transparent on exposure to the air, melts when acted upon by heat, and has then the odor and smoke of meat while roasting. It is particularly nutritious, and is assimilated and digested with facility. If blood is allowed to remain still for a short time in an open vessel, it separates into two parts; the heaviest portion, or that which remains at the bottom, is the fibrine; the remainder, lighter, liquid and transparent, is called the serum; and

Albumen exists in serum. It is insipid and inodorous, soluble in cold water, and passes at once to the state of putrefaction, when exposed in a moist state to the atmosphere. It is coagulated by hot water, and distinguished by this character from all other animal fluids. From its coagulability, it is of great use in clarifying liquids. The white of eggs consists almost wholly of pure albumen.

Gelatine forms the principal proportion of tendinous, cartilaginous substance, exists in all cellular membrane, and predominates in the flesh of very young animals. It is soluble in hot water, and assumes, on cooling, an elastic, tremulous consistence; that form known as "jelly." The "portable soup," which is carried to sea, and preserved in the shape of solid cakes for several years, is prepared by boiling any animal substance, clarifying the liquid with albumen, evaporating to a thick paste, and afterwards drying by heat. It is precipitated, in an insoluble form, by tannin; and it is this action of tannin on gelatine that gives rise to the process of preparing leather for the various purposes to which the latter is applied. Gelatine is nutritious and readily digested.

Oil, or fat, is nutritious, nearly the whole being assimilated; but it is, as has been before stated, very difficult of digestion, experiencing little change, until it has been acted upon by the bile. In the experiments undertaken upon the free gastric secretion, obtained by Dr. Beaumont, it was ascertained, that, while the chymification of other alimentary matters took place seasonably, the oily portions were long in undergoing modification.

Caseine is insipid, inodorous, insoluble in water,

but quickly dissolved by alkalies and some acids. It is distinguished from fibrine and albumen by its greater solubility, and by not coagulating when heated. It may be obtained pure from the curd of milk, and constitutes the principal bulk of cheese. Caseine is less digestible and less nutritious than the other principles above noticed.

Osmazome is another element of animal food, imparting to cooked meat its flavor; but it does not exist in quantity sufficiently large to be distinguished as one of the chief principles in such aliment.

It will be sufficient for the present purpose to notice the three principal divisions into which organized animal substances have been ranged, viz. *fibrinous*, *gelatinous*, and *albuminous*.

In the first class, in which *fibrine* predominates, are included mutton, beef, pork, ducks, geese, and venison.

In the *gelatinous* class are included veal, lamb, young poultry, and certain kinds of fish.

In the *albuminous* class are oysters, eggs, roe of fish, brain, liver, and the sweet bread.

"The healthy stomach," says Dr. Paris, "disposes most readily and effectually of solid food, of a certain specific degree of density, which may be termed its *digestive texture:* if it exceeds this, it will require a greater length of time, and more active powers, to complete its chymification; and if it approaches too nearly to a gelatinous condition, the stomach will be equally impeded in its operations. It is perhaps not possible to appreciate or express the exact degree of firmness, which will confer the highest order of digestibility upon food; indeed, this degree may vary in different individuals; but we are taught by experience, that no meat is so digestible as tender *mutton*. When well conditioned, it appears to possess that degree of consistence which is most congenial to the stomach. It will not be difficult," he adds, "to understand why a certain texture and coherence of the aliment should confer upon it digestibility, or otherwise. Its conversion into chyme is effected by the solvent power of the gastric juice, aided by the churning which it undergoes by the motions of the stomach; and, unless the substance introduced possess a suitable degree of firmness, it will not yield to such motions: this is the case with soup and other liquid aliments; in such cases, therefore, nature removes the watery part before digestion can be carried forward. It is on this account that oils are digested with so much difficulty; and it is probable that jellies and other glutinous matters, although containing the elements of nourishment in the highest state of concentration, are not digested without considerable difficulty; in the first place, on account of their evading the grappling powers of the stomach, and, in the next, in consequence of their tenacity opposing the absorption of their more fluid parts. For these reasons, I maintain that the addition of isinglass and other glutinous matter to animal broths, with a view to render them more nutritive to invalids, is a pernicious custom."

DIFFERENT KINDS OF ANIMAL FOOD.

Mutton is, of all meats, the most highly nutritious, the most digestible, and is perhaps the most generally used. *Beef* enables one to bear more fatigue; but it is not so digestible as mutton, and not so well adapted for dyspeptics and other invalids. Both, however, are readily assimilated to the nature of chyme, and hold the highest rank in the dietetic regimen of Hahnemann. The broth made from beef contains less oil, but more osmazome, than that made of mutton, and is therefore better for the convalescent.

Pork is not readily digested, and by no means proper food for the debilitated and sickly. It can only be eaten with impunity by the most robust laborer. It predisposes to diseases of the lymphatic system, occasions cutaneous disorders, and increases any derangement which may exist in the digestive apparatus. *Bacon* is subject to the same objections, though it is somewhat more easy of digestion.

Ducks and *Geese*, in consequence of their oleaginous nature, are indigestible, and oppressive to delicate stomachs.

Venison is digested with uncommon facility, and is very nutritious and wholesome.

Veal is included in the gelatinous class, and is obnoxious to the same objections as those above applied to pork. It has not become sufficiently matured to possess the requisite alimentation. The same may be said of *Lamb*, this meat likewise not having acquired the suitable degree of animalization.

The flesh of all young animals contains more gelatine than the old, and is much more difficult of digestion. It is, however, better adapted, generally, for those who may be disposed to plethora or inflammatory affections. Gelatine is furnished in large quantity from the tendinous portions of the animal. If broth is to be made from either veal or lamb, — although, in all cases, beef and mutton are to be preferred for this purpose, — the boiling should be continued sufficiently long for the extraction of all the gelatine; and this is to be determined by the liquid, on cooling, readily assuming the consistence of thick jelly.

Of a character neither decidedly fibrinous nor gelatinous, but participating in both, is the flesh of poultry and of certain fish. The fibres, though differing in appearance, are of the nature of beef, mutton, &c. while gelatine largely abounds in the interstitial spaces. Poultry differs in its alimentary properties according as it is young and gelatinous, or old and more fibrinous. That of middle age is the most suitable for invalids. The wild fowl is also preferable to those reared upon farms. The sea-fish usually contains more gelatine than the fish taken from fresh water.

Those articles of food classed as albuminous are, in general, nourishing and readily digested. It will be seen, from Dr. Beaumont's experiments, that the *egg*, when boiled soft, digests half an hour sooner than when boiled hard, and that the raw egg is more digestible than that which is cooked. When in combination with flour and butter, it is rendered more difficult of digestion, and, in the debilitated, often causes uncomfortable sensations of oppression. Eggs contain much nutritive substance in small bulk, and, when the stimulus of animal food is to be avoided, are, of course, improper. Although the white of the egg is almost purely albuminous, the yolk contains animal oil, and on this account, particularly by certain modes of preparation, as in frying, may be rendered very indigestible.

Oysters are nutritious, and of all shell-fish the most digestible, especially if eaten uncooked. The different methods of preparing them for the table, while adding but little to their nutritious qualities, detract much from their digestibility. The liquid by which they are surrounded in the shell has been affirmed by some old writers to be "equal, in medicinal virtue, to the most accredited mineral waters;"

but no proof can be adduced in favor of such an assertion. The *clam* is not so digestible as the oyster. Other shell-fish, as the mussel, lobster, and crab, are not so easy of digestion, although their nutritient properties may be as great. They sometimes produce gastric derangement, and to certain persons are positively injurious. Many cases of poisoning are on record which have resulted from the eating of different shell-fish.

The flesh of fish resembles that of quadrupeds, containing, however, no osmazome, but consisting of fibrine, albumen, and gelatine. It is not, on the whole, as nutritious; and the comparative digestibility of different kinds of fish depends much upon the quantity of oil which they contain. Those without scales are more oleaginous, and on this account less digestible. Smoked and salted fish, as well as meat thus prepared, are unsuited for those persons whose digestive powers are not in the most vigorous condition. They are among the articles expressly interdicted in the homœopathic regimen for the sick.

VEGETABLE FOOD.

The principal elements of vegetable substances which afford nutrition are *fecula*, *gluten*, *mucilage*, *oil*, and *sugar*.

Fecula, or starch, is white, insipid, insoluble in

cold, but converted into a jelly by hot, water. It is one of the chief constituent parts of most varieties of grain, of the roots, seeds, fruit of certain plants, and forms the principal source of nutriment derived from them. It is generally procured for domestic purposes from wheat and the potato, but may be obtained from acorn or the horse-chestnut. The nutritious properties which abound in arrow-root, sago, and tapioca, depend almost wholly upon the presence of fecula.

Gluten. If the flour of wheat is made into a paste, and washed in water, it separates into three distinct substances, — a saccharine mucilage; starch, which subsides on standing; and gluten, which is tenacious, ductile, elastic, and of a brown-gray color. It resembles animal albumen, being quickly coagulated by heat, and is found in numerous vegetable productions, in rye, barley, beans, peas, &c. but in smaller quantity than in wheat. The tenacious paste made by the mixture of flour with water is owing to the presence of gluten; and this principle produces the sponginess of bread, through the detention, by its viscidity, of the carbonic acid gas, disengaged by the process of fermentation. The whole mass of dough is distended by the detained air. Gluten is similar, in many respects, both to animal fibrine and albumen, and has been termed a vegeto-animal element.

Mucilage, or gum, is common in vegetables, but

is furnished in its purest form from the "Acacia vera," the tree producing what is known as "gum-arabic." It is transparent, of an insipid or slightly saccharine taste, and in combination, in any quantity, with water, forms a more or less viscid solution. It is not, however, strictly soluble. Mucilage, like all the proximate vegetable principles, is very nutritive.

Oil, in the vegetable, is similar in character to that of the animal. It is very abundant in the olive (*olea*), from which it derives its name. It is of an unctuous nature, either solid or fluid, not soluble in water, and more or less volatile. Oil exists in the three kingdoms of nature, — the animal, the vegetable, and the mineral; but originated in the latter from the decomposition of the former, — the remains of animal or vegetable existence.

Sugar is obtained from many plants in great abundance, and is quite nutritious. Its appearance and properties are too well known to require description. Upon its presence depends the vinous and acetous fermentations.

DIFFERENT KINDS OF VEGETABLE FOOD.

Of the farinaceous vegetables, or those esculent productions which are reduced to flour in their preparation for food, and which consist of gluten, mucilage, and starch, *wheat* is the most important, as administering most copiously in the form of bread to man's sustenance. It stands first among the "cerealia" of bromatologists. Indian corn, rye, barley, oats, rice, and the buckwheat, are also among the cereal productions.

The bread made from the flour of wheat is that which is the most extensively used, and the best adapted for food of all alimentary substances. Its digestibility depends upon many circumstances connected with its preparation. If properly kneaded and baked, it is very nutritious and digestible. "Good bread ought to be composed of fine wheaten flour, well kneaded with pure water, seasoned with a little salt, fermented with good yeast, and sufficiently baked at a proper heat. When baked, it ought to appear through a glass like honeycomb, full of cells, yet the intermediate parts constituting a uniform substance of a gelatinous nature, which readily unites with an aqueous menstruum." A mixture of the bran with the flour renders bread less liable to form a cohesive mass, after imperfect mastication, and, though less nutritious than pure flour, is better suited for torpid habits, on account of the stimulating effects of the bran upon the mucous membrane. The addition of butter and sugar diminishes the digestible properties of bread. That which is made from barley, rye, &c. often becomes acid in the stomach, and gives rise to uncomfortable sensations of oppression. Bread is more wholesome when eaten the day after having been baked. There are many injurious articles, such as potash, alum, magnesia, and sulphate of copper, mixed with the bread made for sale, for the purpose of improving its appearance. Spoiled flour, unwholesome in itself, is frequently made into bread in Europe, — perhaps in this country, — and alum, magnesia, or copper added to give it the appearance of that made from good flour. Such adulterations are extremely prejudicial to health; and the fact that practices of this kind are ever resorted to, should serve as an incitement to the more general use of "household bread."

Rice is the principal aliment of the inhabitants of several eastern countries. It does not contain much saccharine matter, and does not tend to putrefaction or acescency. It is nutritious and digestible.

The *Potato*, in which a large proportion of starch exists, is, when mealy and not overdone, a very nutritive, wholesome article of food. When water is, as far as practicable, excluded, and the cooking is conducted by steam, it is much more digestible as well as palatable. When roasted or baked, it is less indigestible than when boiled. The raw potato has been found useful both as a preventive and a cure for the diseases induced by a long-continued use of animal aliment, particularly the "salted provisions." The sweet potato is as nutritious, though not as digestible, as the common potato.

Among the farinaceous productions selected for

those enfeebled by disease, as being less substantial but bland and nutritious, are macaroni, vermicelli, arrow-root, sago, tapioca, &c. The two former are preparations of fine flour, having the character of light bread. *Arrow-root* is obtained from a species of the "Maranta" herb, cultivated in the West Indies. It contains a large proportion of nourishment. The most pure is that from Bermuda, which is a clear white, tasteless and odorless. *Sago* is procured from the pith of a palm-tree (*Cycas circinalis*) growing in Java, Molucca, and the Philippine Isles, where it is the chief article of food. *Tapioca* is the condensed starch obtained from the root of the "Jatropha Manihot," a Brazilian plant. The root, when in a raw state, is poisonous; but this quality is destroyed by heat. All of the above constitute light and digestible nutriment, especially adapted for that debilitated condition of body, to which much stimulating aliment would be unsuitable and deleterious.

The leguminous vegetables, — beans, peas, &c. — contain much nourishment, but more fecula and oil than farina, and for this reason are not so easy of digestion as those above described. They frequently cause much pain and flatulence. In the dried state, they are digested with difficulty. The bean is wholly unfit for food, except among those whose digestive organs are in the most healthy condition. But few alimentary combinations are so thoroughly indigestible as baked beans, flanked with pork and swimming in fat, — that favorite Sunday-dish of the New Englander.

The succulent roots, as the turnip, carrot, parsnip, and beet, are of small comparative importance as nutrient articles of diet. They possess chiefly saccharine qualities, and are liable to cause heartburn and flatulency, particularly with dyspeptic sufferers. The *beet* consists more of nutriment than either of the others above named. It contains 15 per cent of nutritious substance, 12 per cent of which is saccharine. A large amount of pure sugar is now manufactured from the beet. The fibrous portions of these roots are unchanged by the gastric and other secretions, — of course, are entirely worthless as aliment. The onion, cabbage, asparagus, and squash, contain but little nutriment. The tomato, though not particularly nutritious, is regarded as one of the most wholesome and valuable esculents among vegetable productions. Whenever diseases prevail in which the digestive organs are implicated, the vegetables above mentioned should be abstained from altogether.

Most varieties of fruit are agreeable to the taste, and refreshing; but their nutritious properties are very inconsiderable. The same restrictions should be placed upon them as upon the succulent vegetables, under the circumstances alluded to in the preceding section.

It may be well to remark in conclusion, that the exclusive use of either animal or vegetable food does not appear to be so productive of health, in temperate regions, as a proper combination of both. The organization of the human digestive apparatus, as has been previously stated, favors the view that a mixture of animal with vegetable food is the most natural for man; and, although reference has been repeatedly made by the opponents of animal aliment to the fact that whole nations subsist exclusively upon a vegetable diet, that they are vigorous and healthy in consequence, — yet it can, on the other hand, be proved that the natives of other countries make use altogether of animal food, and that they are equally healthy. The Indian on the western prairies lives upon buffalo meat; the Hindoo, upon rice and water. Certain African tribes subsist upon roots; the Esquimaux, upon fat and oil. The principal, and, in some instances, the exclusive food of the Irish peasant is the potato; and the food of the "Dobenahs" is the flesh of the elephant and ostrich. It appears to be well established, that, under certain influences of climate and habit, not only can human life be supported, but human health can be maintained, by the exclusive use of either animal or vegetable food; that either or both are in accordance with man's nature. Whichever may have been adopted from childhood, or until the system is habituated to it, becomes the most suitable. It is a hazardous experiment for one accustomed to a mixed diet to enter suddenly upon the practice of total abstinence from animal or vegetable food. In either case, as a general consequence, scorbutic affections, if no other, would result. Magendie's experiments demonstrate, that man, in temperate latitudes, absolutely needs the variety of food which is there so bountifully supplied; that, as nature and habit have combined to render him omniverous, he should be content so to remain.

According to the experiments of the distinguished French chemists, MM. Percy and Vaugelin,—

100 lbs.	Lentils . . contain .	94	parts of	nourishment.
„ „	French Beans . . .	92	„	„
„ „	Rice	90	„	„
„ „	Kidney Beans . . .	89	„	„
„ „	Wheat	85	„	„
„ „	Barley	83	„	„
„ „	Good Bread . . .	80	„	„
„ „	Rye	80	„	„
„ „	Meat (average) . .	35	„	„
„ „	Potatoes	25	„	„
„ „	Carrots	14	„	„
„ „	Beets	14	„	„
„ „	Turnips	8	„	„
„ „	Cabbage	7	„	„
„ „	Greens	6	„	„

CHAPTER II.

ON DRINK.

THAT liquid which the Creator has furnished for man in the greatest abundance, making it the basis of all circulating fluids, — the medium by which all vital action is executed, and without which even solid substances would be innutritious, — is the beverage best calculated to allay thirst, to renovate declining strength, to form, develop, and support the system. Water is, in youth as in age, in summer and in winter, in health and in disease, positively, imperiously demanded by Nature for drink, and no other liquid will supply its place, — none other is needed. To fulfil properly its purpose in the animal economy, it should be pure, — free from any foreign admixture. One form in which it is supplied to many dwellers upon earth is by rain; and this is, or would be, were the air through which it passes perfectly clear, the purest kind of water. In consequence of becoming impregnated with various substances and gases floating in the atmosphere, over large towns especially, rain-water is rendered impure, unpalatable, and subject to a spontaneous change, by long keeping. Besides, it acquires no small amount of additional impurity by washing the roofs of houses, sheds, &c. and running through unclean spouts. In the Island of St. Thomas, spring-water being difficult of access, large cisterns are provided for the purpose of containing the rain-water, which, after the subsidence of the foreign matter held in it, is used for, and highly esteemed as, drink by all the inhabitants.

Water, procured from the melting of snow or ice, is equal to rain-water in purity, and decidedly more agreeable to the taste. In northern latitudes, during the winter, thawed snow forms the constant drink of the people. They do not suffer from "goitre,"— an enlargement of the thyroid gland, — which so deforms many inhabitants in Switzerland, and which has been long supposed to arise from the use of snow-water. There is no good reason for believing that either ice or snow-water is in any degree injurious.

Through an artificial process, in imitation of the natural distillation by which rain is furnished, and in consequence of the easy exclusion of all alien substances, water may be obtained in its purest state. There are no solid nor gaseous substances held in solution by distilled water: it is colorless, perfectly transparent, and entirely devoid of taste and smell; leaving no residuum when carefully evaporated, and capable of preservation for a long time. It is used in the preparation of homœopathic medicines, and, as the purest possible menstruum, is preferred for the administration of remedies in solution.

Although the water obtained from wells, lakes, or rivers is generally acknowledged to be sufficiently pure for the preservation of health, a vast amount of foreign material may be detected in it by chemical analysis. The water from rivers is more free from earthy salts than that from wells. The river Seine, which supplies the city of Paris, furnishes water of excellent quality; and it has been ascertained that the great variety of impurities, which are necessarily received by this river, do not contaminate, or alter the character of the water to any perceptible extent. Filtration will effect the removal of most impurities; and no water, which has been procured either from rivers or lakes, should be used for drink until it has been subjected to this purifying process. The motionless, stagnant water of small ponds, liable to be affected by vegetable and animal decomposition going on within and around it, is not only offensive to the taste, but would be, as a drink, ultimately, if not directly, productive of serious consequences. Dr. Dunglison writes, that, "to render the water of marshes and ponds potable, it has been advised to boil them, under the idea that the boiling temperature will render the organic matters innoxious, and disengage the unwholesome gaseous principles which they may contain. To improve them still farther, they may be agitated, so as to restore the air they have lost by boiling, and be then filtered through sand or charcoal. It has been proposed to add to such water a small quantity of chlorine, or of one of the chlorides; but a quantity sufficient to destroy the foulness of the fluid can hardly fail to communicate a taste and smell, disagreeable to most individuals." He also adds that the Chinese never drink water that has not been boiled.

For the sick, as well as for those in health, simple, uncombined water should be preferred. The cruel, mistaken practice of withholding from the helpless sufferer whose throat is parched, and whose whole frame is heated with fever, the draught of water which he urgently craves, is being abolished; and it is now discovered — thanks to the hydropathist — that cold water, which was once expressly interdicted by the medical attendant as extremely hazardous, is best adapted, in most cases of disease, to afford relief, and promote recovery. The needless suffering which, for centuries, has been caused by an obstinate adherence to the groundless prejudice against cold water for the sick, it would be difficult to over-estimate. In alluding to the hydropathist, it may not be presumptuous to express the opinion that the practice of *deluging* a patient with cold water, internally and externally, and on all occasions, — whether nature does or does not demand it, — is almost, if not quite, as irrational as the old, and it is to be hoped the *abandoned*, custom above referred to. When a sufficiency of water has been drank to administer to the existing necessities of the system, it will be plainly indicated by the patient's sensations. A feeling of satiety evinces as decidedly, after drinking water as after eating food, that enough, or more than enough, has been taken.

The beverages which, next to water, are the most generally used, and which are entitled to the fullest consideration, not only for their dietetic importance, but also for their medicinal properties, are *Coffee* and *Tea;* either or both of which are drank daily by nearly every individual in the country.

COFFEE

Is the fruit of a tree originating in Arabia Felix and Ethiopia, now cultivated in many parts of Europe and America. The berry is at first green in color, afterwards red, and finally dark brown, and is composed of two demi-ovoid hard grains, enveloped with a kind of paper-like membrane. That which comes from Mocha, in Arabia, is of the best quality. Its peculiar principle is cafeine, which is white, volatile, and crystallizable, containing a large quantity of nitrogen; and it has been discovered to be identical with "theine," the bitter principle of tea. Coffee is, to a certain extent, nutritious, and the addition of sugar and milk renders it more so; but its injurious effects upon the nervous system — the evil consequences, in other respects, resulting from its constant use — more than counterbalance all the advantages which have been attributed to it. Possessing narcotic properties, it may be regarded to that degree as poisonous; and no article whatever of such a nature can be introduced continually into the system, without, sooner or later, and in some definite form, affecting health. Its action as a medicine, administered in homœopathic doses, in subduing restlessness, promoting sleep, relieving certain kinds of fevers, counteracting the morbid consequences of certain mental emotions, &c. is undeniable. The strongest opiate is not more decided in soporific influence. Hahnemann pursued his investigations carefully with respect to coffee; and, as the subject is of much importance, we will translate in full from Jourdan's edition the remarks of the author in regard to its effects upon the human system. To aid in acquiring a clear comprehension of the true action of this narcotic, some prefatory observations are made which, in connection with the body of the treatise, we venture to present to the reader. Hahnemann thus writes: —

"For the prolongation of life, and for the preservation of health, man should make use of aliment which is simply nutritive, and which contains nothing either irritating or medicinal. His drink should be of a moistening and nutritious character only, like pure water and milk.

"No seasoning to stimulate the palate should be taken other than salt, sugar, and vinegar,—and these three in small quantities, since in this way they cannot materially injure. All of the so-called 'sweetmeats,' and all spirituous drinks, partake, more or less, of the nature of medicine. The nearer they approach the medicinal,—the more frequently they are introduced into the stomach, and the greater the quantity taken,—in the same proportion are they injurious to health, and tend to the shortening of life.

"The greatest danger consists in making habitual use of purely medicinal substances, which possess strong active qualities.

"Wine was the only drink purely medicinal among the ancients; but the Greeks and Romans were wise enough never to drink without copiously *watering* their wine. In modern times, many other medicinal substances, both liquid and solid, have been introduced into diet. Tobacco is smoked, chewed, and stuffed into the nostrils; opium is eaten; spirituous and malt liquors drank; tea and coffee used in excess.

"Medicinal substances are those which do not nourish, but which injure the health. Every thing which injures health is contrary to nature,—a kind of disease. That which is medicinal has the power of annihilating the unnatural condition which is called disease, in proportion to the power which it possesses of producing disease in the healthy body. Except in case of disease, medicines are injurious. To make frequent use of them, to introduce them into dietetic regimen, is to destroy the harmony of the organs, to diminish health, and to abridge life.

"Coffee is a substance almost entirely medicinal.

"All medicines given in large doses exercise an injurious influence upon a healthy person. No one can smoke tobacco without experiencing, for the first time, great aversion. No one finds pure coffee without sugar agreeable the first time it is taken. This is a caution which nature gives us not to violate the laws of health, — not to trample under foot the instinct which was given as the preserver of health and life.

"If, yielding to fashion and to example, medicinal substances continue to be used, habit blunts, by degrees, the disagreeable impression which they at first produce upon us. They end often by giving pleasure; that is to say, the apparently agreeable action which they exercise upon our organs becomes insensibly a necessity for us.

"It so happens also, that, having been brought to a certain degree, into an unhealthy condition by medicinal substances, instinct leads us to continue the use of them, to comfort us, momentarily at least, by the palliative influence which they exert upon the inconveniences of which they are, from time to time, the source. To comprehend this, it will be necessary to understand that every thing medicinal produces two opposing effects upon the human body. Its primitive effect is precisely the reverse of the secondary effect, — that is, the state in which the body is left many hours after the primitive effect has ceased.

"Most medicines occasion among those in health disagreeable and painful sensations, which, during the secondary effect, are the reverse of those which exist during the primitive effect; and even their prolonged use never produces agreeable impressions upon him who is in health.

"The primitive effect of coffee consists, generally, in a more or less agreeable exaltation of the vital energy. The animal functions, natural and vital, as they are named, are artificially excited by it at first. But the secondary effect, which manifests itself afterwards little by little, brings about a totally opposite state; that is, an unhappy sense of existence, an ebbing of life, a kind of paralysis of the animal functions, natural and vital.

"When one not accustomed to coffee takes it in moderation, or when one habituated to this beverage uses it in excess, he experiences, for the first few hours, a vivid sense of his own existence. His pulse is more full, more frequent, but more feeble. A circumscribed redness is seen upon the cheeks, which does not extend by insensible degrees, but shows like a stain. The forehead and the palms of the hands are covered with a moisture. More warmth is felt than before, and this sensation produces a pleasurable uneasiness. The heart is agitated by agreeable palpitations. The veins of the hands become swollen. A more than ordinary heat of the skin is perceived by the touch; but this heat never becomes burning, even after a strong dose of coffee, and it soon terminates in a general perspiration. The presence of mind and the faculty of attention are as active as in the ordinary state. Every object appears to wear a smiling aspect. For the first few hours, the coffee-drinker is contented with himself, and with all who surround him. It is this which has elevated coffee to the rank of a social drink.

"When the primitive effect has passed, the opposite condition gradually appears, which is the secondary effect or re-action. The more decided the first, the more pronounced and disagreeable will be the second.

"The abuse of this medicinal beverage causes more inconveniences in some than in others.

"Our bodies are organized with an art so admirable, that slight errors in diet do not greatly injure us, while we are living in other respects a life conformable to nature. Thus, for example, the German laborer drinks every morning a certain quantity of brandy; and, if the quantity be small, it does not prevent him from arriving often at quite an advanced age. His health suffers but little; for his good constitution, and the salubrious mode of life which he otherwise leads, counteracts the evil influences of such a practice. If, instead of brandy, he should take every morning one or two cups of coffee, the result would be the same. The vigor of his frame, the active exercise to which he is subjected, and the abundance of pure air which he every day respires, weaken the influence of the beverage, and his health does not apparently suffer.

"But the injurious effects of coffee are much more decided upon those who are not placed in such favorable circumstances.

"The man who passes his life confined to his house or room may enjoy a sort of health, when he follows a regimen in other respects appropriate to his situation. If he is temperate, if he makes use of easily-digested food, if he confines himself to simple drinks, if he controls his appetites and passions, and if he frequently renews the air in his apartment, he may, on these conditions, enjoy a certain degree of health, which, it is true, may be affected by the slightest cause, but which is none the less a source of relative well-being. The action of all morbific influences, of all medicines, for example, is much more evident and powerful upon such persons, than upon those who are robust and accustomed to work in the open air, who can endure pernicious impressions without much comparative injury.

"When, at the end of a certain period, the primitive action of coffee, that is to say, the factitious exaltation of the vital activity, is dissipated, a desire to sleep comes on, accompanied by inertia greater than usual. Motion is disagreeable, cheerfulness disappears, and is succeeded by a sad and morose humor. The agreeable sensation of warmth is no longer felt, the least variation of temperature causes disagreeable sensations, and the hands, as well as the feet, become cold. External objects are viewed under a less flattering aspect. A sort of craving, promptly satisfied, replaces the natural appetite; and, while food and drink oppress the stomach, the head becomes heavy. The sleep is unrefreshing; the awaking, difficult and painful.

"But, in the morning, a fresh resort to the injurious palliative removes for a while the evil, and again a factitious energy commences; enduring, however, a shorter length of time than at first. The coffee must be taken more frequently, or stronger, as is the case with opium and alcohol, until a tolerable degree of energy is acquired. And thus, day after day, the constitution of the sedentary man deteriorates. The surface of the body grows more sensitive, not only to cold, but to the influence of fresh air, whatever may be its temperature; digestion is accomplished in a laborious manner; sleep is not quiet and profound, but a drowsiness which does not re-animate or refresh. Serenity, cheerfulness, vigor of mind, is changed to timidity, indecision, apathy, sadness; and the mind and body vacillate unceasingly between high excitement and deep depression.

"It would be difficult to describe all the derangements with which coffee-drinkers are affected under the name of nervous diseases.

"It must not be supposed, however, that all who drink coffee experience, in an equal degree, the consequences above described. Such is not the case. With some, a particular symptom is more decided; while, with others, a different symptom of the secondary effect is more obvious. My description embraces all classes of coffee-drinkers, and I mention those symptoms only which are fairly attributable to the source in question.

"The agreeable sensation of increased energy which coffee causes for a time, gives place, on the occasion of the secondary action, to many uncomfortable feelings, which are augmented in proportion to the strength and frequency of the draughts. A slight influence which would produce no impression upon one in health and unaccustomed to coffee, gives rise, in one who uses it, to headaches, frequent pain in the teeth, often insupportable, recurring especially at night, and sharp pains in different parts of the body. Erysipelatous affections not unfrequently arise from this cause. Restlessness, feverish heat, nervous headaches, constantly disturb the coffee-drinker. No impropriety in regimen occasions more readily and more certainly caries of the teeth than the use of coffee, unless it be that of mercury. The incisive teeth are those most quickly affected.

"In general, coffee exercises a most pernicious influence upon children, and so much the more as they are more delicate. After children, women and literary men are more injured, inasmuch as their occupations oblige them to lead sedentary lives. To this class may be added craftsmen who are shut up in their workshops.

"Certain persons, led in some sort by instinct, find in spirituous liquors a kind of antidote to coffee. It cannot be denied that these drinks exert this counteracting effect to a certain extent. But they are merely new irritants, without any nutritive properties; that is to say, medicinal substances, which, when taken daily, will bring on other inconveniences, without removing those of the coffee. They are fresh exciting impulses to life, leaving in their train evils of a different and yet more complicated nature.

"The principal means of removing the evil consequences of coffee is, after renouncing the drink, to exercise actively in the open air. But, if the mind and body are too much enfeebled for the adoption of this course, it will then be necessary to have recourse to appropriate medicines, which will not be here designated, since this treatise is not for such a purpose designed.

"Supported by a long experience, I do not hesitate to declare that the daily use of coffee is a most pernicious practice, and as one of the surest methods of weakening and ultimately destroying all mental and physical energy. This drink has been termed medicinal, and it may be said that medicines are salutary. No medicine can be useful to a man in health, and no man can be healthy who makes frequent use of medicine.

"It must be admitted that coffee facilitates digestion in some cases; and, when gastric and intestinal inaction or torpidity exists, it may be temporarily beneficial. But the salutary effects attributed to coffee, and by which those who take much of it seek to justify the habit which they have contracted, are reduced almost entirely to palliative results. Now, a fact admitting of no dispute is this, that, if the prolonged use of any palliative remedy whatever causes injury to health, nothing can be more pernicious than such a substance among the articles of *daily* consumption.

"While opposing the use of coffee as an habitual drink, I nevertheless estimate highly its medicinal virtues, both as a curative remedy in the chronic diseases, the symptoms of which bear a great resemblance to the primitive effects, or as a palliative remedy in the rapidly developed and imminently dangerous affections whose symptoms greatly resemble the secondary effects of this narcotic. These are the only cases benefited by a medicinal substance, which millions of men make use of to their own great detriment, the true value of which few know, and which exerts a most salutary influence where it is properly administered."

Such is the opinion of one who had thoroughly studied the properties of coffee; and, however exaggerated the account of its action may appear to many, daily observation confirms its truth. That it has been partaken of by some as a daily beverage, without perceptible injury, throughout the course of a long life, is no better argument in favor of its general use than is the same argument when applied to the habitual use of alcohol.

It may be well to remark here, for the benefit of those who are wedded to this drink, that, when a large proportion of milk is added to coffee, the deleterious effects of the latter are, to a considerable extent, neutralized, and the degree of harmless nutriment obtained from this addition of milk makes the beverage much less objectionable. The French prepare the berry with great nicety, neither charring nor slightly roasting it, and add to the decoction one-half, or more, of boiled milk. In this form, it is drank with comparative impunity. Volney, while travelling, several years since, through the United States, observed that the Americans hastily swallowed large quantities of a strong, nauseous, and muddy decoction, which they called "coffee;" and, what with their hurried manner of "bolting" half-cooked food at the same time, it was not very surprising that *dyspepsia* should be so prevalent in this country.

TEA.

This plant is a native of China, and, though dignified with the name of tree, seldom attains the height of more than five feet. Its leaves are dried upon iron plates, suspended over a fire, and afterwards packed in tin boxes for exportation. Although a very large amount of these leaves are shipped to Europe and America, it has been asserted, that, were the commerce wholly abandoned, the price of tea would not be much lessened in China, so great is the domestic consumption. In the year 1838, there were imported into Great Britain 32,366,412 pounds of this article. In this country more than 16,000,000 pounds are now annually received and consumed. The class designated by the term "green" includes hyson, young hyson, imperial gunpowder, and hyson skin. The "black" teas are the bohea, pouchong, souchong, &c.

With respect to the nutritive properties of tea, analysis shows that, out of 100 parts, 84 are tannin, and woody fibre; 6 are gluten; and 6 are mucilage; the remaining 4 parts consisting of volatile matter, &c. Thus it will be perceived, that, without the addition of sugar and milk, its nutrient properties are small. Tannin constitutes about 40 in 100 parts. This is well known to be an astringent principle, consequently acting as a medicinal power upon the system. It tends to combine with gelatine, as has been before stated, forming an insoluble compound; and, of course, from this chemical action, must render whatever gelatine it may meet with in the stomach indigestible. The green teas are found to be more astringent than the blacks. They are more narcotic, and, on account of their greater medicinal qualities, are prohibited during homœopathic treatment; while the black teas, much diluted with water, are permitted to be used.

Tea, made strong and drank frequently, produces consequences upon the nervous system almost as serious as those from coffee. Its effects are like those of all narcotic poisons. Though their action may be upon some temperaments scarcely perceptible for a time, they are none the less certain to bring on, eventually, derangements, similar to those enumerated by Hahnemann as produced by coffee; such as nervous headaches, tremors, mental depression, &c.

The same observations which were made with reference to coffee, as a palliative, are applicable to tea. By its diluent and sedative influence, it may impart relief in many cases of irritability dependent on febrile action. It alleviates headache; but the result is effected by virtue of the power which it possesses of producing headache, through its action upon the nervous system.

Although, like coffee, it is useless to deny that tea possesses useful qualities, it is only as a medicine that it acts favorably; — and, whatever may be the kind or the strength used, it is still a medicine; — and the impropriety of taking daily any article of a medicinal nature has been made sufficiently obvious by the investigations of Hahnemann.

In the Appendix to "Pereira's Treatise," edited by Dr. Lee, are the following remarks respecting the article under consideration: "Green tea undoubtedly possesses very active medicinal properties; for a very strong decoction of it, or the extract, *speedily destroys life* in the inferior animals, *even when given in very small doses.* This has been repeatedly tested by experiment, and may therefore be taken as an undoubted fact. The strongly marked effects of tea upon persons of a highly nervous temperament, in causing wakefulness, tremors, palpitations, and other distressing feelings, prove also that it is an agent of considerable power, and should not be used to any great extent by persons of such a habit. It not unfrequently occasions vertigo and sick headache, together with a sinking sensation at the pit of the stomach, shortly after eating. It is also opposed to an active nutrition, and should therefore be used with great moderation by those who are very thin in flesh. From its astringent properties, it is often useful in certain conditions; and, from its pleasurable, exhilarating effects, it is often recommended to the studious, the sedentary, and those affected with low spirits and indigestion. We are, however, satisfied that green tea does not, in any case, form a salubrious beverage for persons in health, and should give place to milk, milk and water, black tea, milk and sugar, which, taken tepid, form very agreeable and healthy drinks."

CHOCOLATE, MILK, WHEY, ETC.

Chocolate is prepared from the nut of the cacao-tree, a native of the West Indies. The kernels of the nut, after being heated upon an iron plate, and afterwards ground, form, with the addition of water, a paste, which is sweetened, flavored, dried in moulds of different shapes, and sold in the shops as chocolate. Cocoa is a preparation of the same substance, — the husks, as well as the kernels, being ground up together. Both are nutritious as beverages, more so than tea or coffee, and do not contain any strictly medicinal properties; but the large proportion of oil which enters into their composition renders them indigestible, and therefore unsuitable for those whose digestive powers are enfeebled. If the oil of the nut is extracted, the indigestibility is of course diminished; and the "prepared cocoa," which contains but little oil, is the least objectionable for invalids. As a daily beverage, however, both chocolate and cocoa are much to be preferred to tea or coffee; and, if the process of digestion and assimilation proceed in a healthy manner, they cannot be productive of any injurious results.

Milk occupies a middle rank between vegetable and animal food. While not strictly a beverage, it is chiefly used as such by the adult. It has been considered by some as of a purely vegetable nature; but it surely is erroneous thus to class it, since it is manifestly absurd to call the milk taken for instance from a carniverous animal a vegetable production. It contains saccharine, oleaginous, aqueous, and albuminous ingredients, — four principles, to which Dr. Prout reduced all alimentary matters. The aqueous principle, which forms so large a portion of all organized substances, constitutes nearly nine-tenths of milk. Dr. Prout regarded fibrine, gluten, and gelatine as modifications of albumen; classed all vegetable principles under the head of saccharine; animal and vegetable oils under that of the oleaginous. He says that the composition of the substances by which animals are usually nourished, favors the mixture of the primary staminal alimentary principles; since most of these substances are compounds of at least two of the staminal principles. Thus, most of the gramineous and herbaceous matters contain the saccharine or amylaceous and the glutinous principles; while every part of an animal contains at least albumen (assuming here its general identity with fibrine) and oil. Perhaps, therefore, it is impossible to name a substance constituting the food of the more perfect animals, which is not essentially a natural compound of at least two, if not all the three, great principles of aliment. But it is in the artificial food of man that we see this great principle of mixture strongly exemplified. He, dissatisfied with the spontaneous productions of nature, culls from every source; and by the force of his reason, or rather of his instinct, forms in every possible manner, and under every disguise, the same great alimentary compound. This, after all his cooking and his art, how much soever he may be disinclined to believe it, is the sole object of his labor; and the more nearly his results approach to this object, the more nearly do they approach perfection. Even in the utmost refinements of luxury, and in his choicest delicacies, the same great principle is attended to; and his sugar and flour, his eggs and butter, in all their various forms and combinations, are nothing more or less than disguised imitations of the great alimentary prototype, *milk*, as furnished to him by nature.

Milk is the natural food of the young of all animals of the mammalia class, and contains all the nutritious qualities necessary for their sustenance; but it is not to be inferred, in consequence, that it will prove sufficient for the adult animal. It is more nutritive than vegetable, and less so than animal, food. Many persons cannot be restricted to a milk diet without suffering from acescency, and other symptoms of indigestion; and, in certain morbid affections, it appears to be entirely unsuitable. As an additional proof that a diet exclusively vegetable was not originally intended for man, it may be stated that human milk is less abundant, thinner, and more acidulous, and for this reason not so well adapted for the support of the child, when the mother lives entirely on vegetable food. In this connection, it is well to add that the milk is readily affected, not only by the kind of aliment taken, but by mental emotions, and especially by medicinal substances. The injurious consequences of medicine in large doses and in a crude state, administered at times so copiously to nursing mothers, are not confined to them, but act most sensibly upon the impressible system of the infant, through the medicated secretion of milk; and the helpless young creature is thus forced to draw in poisoned food, even for a long time after the direct medicinal action upon the mother has ceased. So evident is this transmitted influence, that, in order to counteract many morbid conditions in the child, it is oftentimes only necessary to administer the appropriate homœopathic remedy to the mother; which, being absorbed without injury to the latter, is conveyed through the medium of the food to the little patient.

Whey is the watery and least nutritious part of milk, freed, in a great measure, from the caseous and butyraceous properties; and from the absence, or greatly diminished amount, of these qualities, it is better adapted as a beverage for the sick, and especially in febrile, acute diseases.

Buttermilk is milk which has been deprived of its oleaginous portion by agitation. When milk has been preserved but a short time before this separation is made to take place, the buttermilk is less acidulous than if the milk has been long kept before the butter is separated. In consequence of the removal of the oily matter, it is more digestible than pure milk, although less nutritive, and, for this reason, is better fitted as a beverage in inflammatory and other diseases. It is refrigerant in proportion to its acidity, but this renders the drink liable to produce gastric inconveniences.

Sugar of Milk is the saline substance obtained from the whey by evaporation. It has also been termed the "essential salt of milk." That which is sold in this country is usually procured from Switzerland, where it is prepared from the whey, there existing in large quantities during the preparation of cheese. As a non-medicinal vehicle, sugar of milk is much used in the trituration and administration of homœopathic medicines, being purified, for this purpose, from all foreign salts.

ALCOHOLIC DRINKS.

Of these artificial liquors there is a great variety, the quantity of alcohol varying, more or less, in each; but they are all, without an exception, injurious to the animal economy. Water is the only fluid which is appointed by nature for human necessities, the most efficient and only suitable diluent or refrigerant; and it certainly is unnecessary and unwise to resort to any other. The most commendable crusade ever undertaken against any of the diabolical agencies which obstruct man's path to heaven, is that now being carried on against the arch-enemy to human health and happiness, — alcohol; the accursed thing that man himself has taken pains to extract from the naturally harmless gifts of God. Certain medical authors have attempted to stigmatize the most blessed movement of the present age, — that of uncompromising opposition to alcohol as a beverage, and have asserted that the temperate use of wine, &c. is not injurious to a healthy person. The course of reasoning adopted to prove this assertion must be of a singular nature. No one in health needs stimulants. They may be of benefit in imparting temporary vigor to the debilated; although Hahnemann, as well as others, has demonstrated that the excitement and strength produced by artificial means is certain to be followed by a corresponding state of depression and debility; and, to avoid the recoil, continued stimulation is required, until it becomes a necessity. "The last state of the man is worse than the first." A morbid appetite is created for that which does not nourish, and cannot become assimilated with, the body. As a beverage, however, alcohol is here to be referred to; and as such, in all its forms, no opposition to it can be too strenuous and persevering.

It is said to be fallacy of reasoning to argue against the *use* of an article from its *abuse*. But, in this instance, one term implies the other. The *use* of any solid or fluid not necessary for sustenance, and for the perservation of health, may be termed its abuse ; but this alcoholic principle, in any shape whatever, is not only needless, but positively inimical to the natural operation of the living functions. It is an absolute poison when pure, and but a diluted poison when weakened ; and, while no one but a madman would attempt to swallow it undiluted, many gradually insinuate the poison into their systems by the more palatable and rather less excoriating form, deluding themselves into the belief that the poison is altogether neutralized by being diluted. It matters not in what shape the " enemy is put into the mouth," even if in not sufficient force at once " to steal away the brains ; " it still remains an enemy, and no " ingenious device " can possibly deprive it of that character. " It [alcohol] does not form a constituent part of any tissue or of any fluid in the healthy body ; it retards, in place of aiding, those series of changes which the aliment undergoes before it is converted into blood ; it is perturbating always, and deleterious generally, to the functions, whether they be merely of nutrition, or those by which man is enabled to speculate on his own situation, and to fulfil his higher destiny." (Dr. Bell on Regimen.)

Alcohol is the product of the vinous fermentation. Having been first obtained from the juice of the grape, it was denominated "spirits of wine." By distillation, or that process by which the volatile are separated, through heat, from the fixed principles, alcohol is procured in its purest state. It exists in different proportions in all intoxicating liquids. To enter into details respecting the comparative amount of alcohol present in the different drinks which pass under the name of rum, brandy, gin, porter, &c. would be unnecessary. It may be sufficient here to state that they contain, in a greater or less degree, the poison which produces morbid changes upon the stomach and brain, and are, one and all, totally unfit for beverages.

Were alcohol a principle which benefited, in place of injuring; improved digestion, instead of disturbing it; elevated man towards the angel, instead of debasing him below the brute, — still the abominable adulterations to which it is, in every saleable form, subjected, ought to exclude it from use. *Wines* are adulterated by lime, alum, lead, corrosive sublimate, and arsenic. Impure when imported, — since the United States is the market for the poorest kinds of wine, — they are doubly so when consumed. *Beer* contains more *quassia* than hops; and the fine froth, which is so strangely attractive, is generally the production of a vile mixture of green vitriol, alum, and salt. *Porter* frequently contains the "cocculus Indicus," a berry brought from Malabar, which is exceedingly poisonous. *Lead* can often be detected in brandy, by slowly boiling until the alcohol has evaporated; and so with the others. There are but few which do not contain a poison, superadded to that they legitimately possess, which alone ought to satisfy the morbid cravings of the irrational, self-abandoned toper.

CHAPTER III.

ON AIR.

The character of the air by which man is surrounded, and which fills the lungs at every inspiration, must of necessity exert a very important influence upon his health. Its density and rarity, its dryness and humidity, its sudden alternations of temperature, its vitiation by emanations from animal and vegetable life, its electric conditions, &c. produce impressions upon the human economy more or less direct and powerful. When it is recollected that there are between 28,000 and 29,000 inspirations in twenty-four hours, and that, during this period, more than one million cubic inches of air are inspired into the lungs for the purpose of rendering the blood which circulates through the entire frame fit for the support of life, the influence of any cause which may detract from the purity of this fluid so essential to existence must be obviously deleterious.

The oxygen of the air, which constitutes one-fifth part of the whole, is indispensable to respiration; the remaining four-fifths is nitrogen or azote, an element destructive to life. Carbonic acid, and other gases which emanate from different substances upon the earth, exist in the atmosphere; but in proportions so inconsiderable to the whole mass, as to be considered rather as heterogeneous and accidental, than as forming any of its component parts. The only ingredient in air which, by itself, can support life, is oxygen; and even this gas is irrespirable, except in that form of combination which naturally exists, and which is found to be uniform in every part of the atmosphere obtainable for analysis. Although, in the ordinary state of air, carbonic acid, which destroys life more rapidly than nitrogen, forms but a very small portion, viz. 1 in 1000 parts, and is, of course, innoxious in this connection, yet it may, under certain circumstances, greatly exceed this proportion; and, while most other deleterious matters prove their existence to the sense of smell, carbonic acid gas may extinguish life, without yielding any premonitory indication of its presence.

It is well known, that, during respiration, the character of the air inspired is altered; that a portion of the oxygen, uniting with the carbon which it meets in the lungs, is converted into carbonic acid; that this carbonic acid is expelled at every expiration, its quantity being the same in amount with that of the oxygen which has disappeared. The nitrogen undergoes no perceptible alteration. It has already been stated by what means carbon is received into the circulation, before forming its combination with oxygen in the lungs. As oxygen is constantly consumed in this manner, and its place in the air supplied by carbonic acid, it is manifest that, without proper caution, health, in a climate which compels much confinement within doors, is continually subject to derangement from the invisible influence which is everywhere present. Ventilation, or the obtaining a plentiful supply of fresh air for apartments where human beings congregate, is a subject to which attention should be especially directed; and, in a hygienic point of view, is of the highest possible interest.

Deteriorated air is one chief cause of the production, or rather the development, of many serious affections. The rise and progress of "scurvy" is believed to be owing, in a greater measure than is generally supposed, to the vitiated air which abounds in the interior of vessels which are not supplied with suitable means of ventilation. The food to which seamen are usually restricted, is, undoubtedly, the primary exciting cause of this disorder; but that its ravages would be greatly limited by an abundance of pure air is not to be denied. In some of the large manufacturing establishments of England, where the air is quite impure, "scrofula" and "rickets" are very common; and, although many other injurious influences, to which disease may be attributed, are at work upon the operatives, still the confined air which they are compelled to breathe, tends materially to elicit the above-named disorders, where a predisposition exists. Scrofula, particularly, is found to be prevalent among the lower classes who reside in the crowded dwellings situate in narrow, confined streets of cities. Baudeloque affirms that "impure air is the true, perhaps the only, cause of scrofulous disease: wherever we find scrofula, that cause exists; where it exists, we find scrofula; and where it is absent, scrofula is not known." Carmichael states, in his small work on scrofula, that this disease prevailed to an extraordinary extent in the House of Industry at Dublin; and that, in one room, 60 feet by 18, with a low ceiling, one hundred and fourteen children were confined through the night and nearly all the day. "When the door of this ward-room was opened in the morning, the air was insupportable."

At the Lying-in Hospital of Dublin, it is stated by Dr. Clarke, that, in 1781, owing to the impurity of the air in the wards, every *sixth* child died, within nine days after birth, of convulsions; and that, after means of thorough ventilation had been adopted, the mortality in the five succeeding years was reduced to nearly 1 in 20. Sir James Clarke also believes that "living in an impure atmosphere is even more influential in deteriorating health than defective food, and that the immense mortality among children and in workhouses is ascribable more to the former than to any other cause. Dr. Combe, in his "Treatise on the Management of Infancy," thus writes: "Those whose attention has never been specially directed to the subject can have no idea of the extent to which this cause (impure air) of bad health in the young is left in operation among even the middle classes of society, and much more from ignorance than any unavoidable necessity. I have seen many examples of this; but the most striking which I have met with was in a very large family, in which scrofula raged with an intensity almost exactly proportioned to the degree of vitiation of the air in which its several members lived. The first-born children escaped altogether, because, in their day, the nursery and bed-rooms were, of course, least crowded, and it was easier to have the occupants much in the open air; but afterwards, when five or six young people, and the nursery-maids, lived and slept in one room of very moderate dimensions, in which cooking and washing were carried on, and two more in a small ill-aired bed-closet adjoining, every one of them suffered severely from the disease. The bad air not being suspected to have any share in the result, no attempt was made to improve it by adequate ventilation, even during the day; and, in consequence, all the medical treatment and means resorted to served only to retard the progress of the scrofula, but without being able to cure it. In this way, the younger members of the family suffered under it for several years; and, in a large proportion of them, it was either directly or indirectly the cause of death. If one-half of the expense incurred for medical attendance and sea-bathing had been devoted from the first to removing the original cause, and procuring a permanent supply of fresh air, a vast amount of anxiety and suffering might have been saved to all, and to none more than to the fond parents, who could only mourn over a fatality which they never imagined it possible to prevent."

Vitiated air impairs the quality of the blood; and, if immediate consequences are not observed to follow confinement in it, it is nevertheless certain that the health will be more or less affected, that the constitution will be undermined, and a foundation laid for diseases which will eventually appear in force, and perhaps result in death years afterward. The air of small rooms or shops, where one or more persons are always present, must be impure, unless a fresh supply is frequently admitted. It should not be supposed, because one does not suffer direct inconvenience, that the air is of sufficiently good quality for respiration. Small apartments, heated during cold weather by a "red-hot demon of a stove," with the chimney blocked up, and every crack and crevice in windows and doors stuffed with wool, are better adapted for the dead than for the living; and, in sleeping apartments, where pure air is especially needed, great care is exercised in excluding it, as though it were an enemy instead of a friend. Is it surprising that indisposition is so often complained of in the morning? If lassitude, drowsiness, inanimation, cannot be accounted for, in such cases, by the inmates of a poisoned bedroom, let them leave it for a moment after rising, and, on their re-entrance, they will be at no loss for a cause. There may be oxygen enough left, it is true, to sustain life; but there is much more carbonic acid and other impurities than is suitable for healthy respiration. It was a sad change, and a most questionable modern improvement, when the open, capacious, ventilating fire-places of a former age gave place to "air-tight stoves" in air-tight apartments.

In the "Grotto del Cano," kingdom of Naples, there has long been an accumulation of carbonic acid gas, which, on account of its greater density, occupies the lower portions of the cave. This is a hole in the side of a mountain near the lake Agnano, measuring not more than eighteen feet from its entrance to the inner extremity. Dogs are there kept for the benefit of the curious traveller, that he may have the rare opportunity of witnessing the immediate and deadly effects of this gas. One of these animals is thrust in by the sordid scoundrel in attendance, and, on being forced to inhale the carbonic acid, it instantly expires; though it is often resuscitated in order to go through subsequent experiments of the same cruel description. Such is the noxious gas exhaled from the human lungs; and, were a person to be enclosed in a perfectly tight box, all external air being completely excluded, he would, as soon as the oxygen was exhausted, cease to exist, suffocated by the carbonic acid which his own breathing had generated. Thus it will be readily perceived, that, by preventing all entrance of pure air into an inhabited room, a poison is unceasingly accumulating, which, though it may continue in a diluted state for a long time, and never perhaps become sufficiently concentrated to produce instant death, is still a poison; acting like the daily draughts of a weakened narcotic, gradually to reduce the vital energy, and prepare the way for the approach of disease and death.

The vicissitudes of temperature, sudden alternations of heat and cold so frequent in our climate, are exciting causes of much disease. The system may accommodate itself after a time to the endurance of either extreme of temperature; for the human race are capable of enjoying a certain degree of health in the intense cold of the frigid zone, as well as under the burning sun of the equator. But when the atmospheric changes are rapid, when the system is kept in a state of constant perturbation and fluctuation, no period of sufficient length intervening to enable it to call up all its powers of resistance to the unexpected agency, a derangement of healthy action must be the consequence. If the alteration is from heat to cold, the cutaneous transpiration, which, as the great depurating medium, should be uninterrupted, is checked; a disturbance is induced in the capillary vessels on the surface, which is transferred, through sympathy, to the mucous membrane lining the interior; and thus catarrhs, inflammation of throat, lungs, intestines, &c. are produced. When the reverse is the case, when the variation from sudden cold to heat occurs, a similar irregularity of action results, and internal inflammations are likewise developed. In passing from a heated room, without sufficient protection, into the external air of a winter's day, the body is exposed to the like influences and consequences. The thermometer in the house may indicate 75 to 80 degrees, and the thermometer without may be below zero, yet thousands of imprudent individuals are daily exposing themselves to this extreme transition; stepping at once, as it were, from the torrid zone into the Arctic regions, with but a trifling difference of clothing. Many strong men have thus jumped from their counting-rooms into a sick-bed; and many delicate women have thus danced out of the ball-room into the grave.

Emanations from the earth, in certain localities, are other prolific sources of disease. In the western parts of our country, the air becomes vitiated by "marsh miasmata," which induce fevers of a peculiar type. Much ignorance prevails with regard to the nature of this poison, and much difference of opinion as to its origin; whether it is generated by animal, vegetable, or aqueous decomposition, or by all combined. Certain it is, that intermittent fevers, which are so prevalent in marshy districts, also occur in localities where no miasm from such sources can be produced. Whatever may be the circumstance or combination of circumstances necessary for the production of the variety of intermittents, it is admitted that a moist atmosphere exercises a considerable influence in their promotion.

In respect to the nature of epidemics in general, what is the peculiar atmospheric condition to which their existence may be ascribed, nothing is known with any degree of certainty. Numerous suggestions have been made relative to the causes which give rise to endemic diseases, such as remittent and intermittent fevers, &c. confined to certain districts, as well as to epidemic diseases, such as plague, influenza, cholera, &c. Electric influences, extreme heat and cold, dryness and humidity of the air, and other agencies, have been mentioned as direct causes, and all have been abandoned as universally inapplicable and inadequate. The plague, for example, which has its principal dwelling-place in Egypt, appears to be the effect of no definite cause, or union of causes, which do not equally prevail where there is no plague. The irregular, undefinable movements of the influenza, the equally indeterminate migrations of the cholera, admit of no satisfactory explanation. That an infectious influence, impalpable, invisible, eluding the keenest investigation, *does* exist,—acting with terrific violence upon the human system, and baffling all medicinal measures of a gross, material nature adopted for its removal,—is undeniable; and while an imperceptible cause is thus in operation, forcing an acknowledgment from all of its immense and unseen power, the similar action of poisons attenuated by art is, *because attenuated*, by the many disregarded, unrecognized, ridiculed, as a delusion of the few.

While referring to unhealthy emanations, it may be well to allude to "intramural interments." It is a subject to which the public attention has been recently directed; and it is "devoutly to be wished," that efficient action may be taken for the immediate abolition of the revolting custom of burying the dead in the very homes of the living. The putrefaction of bodies, crowded into a small space, vitiates the surrounding air; and, as has been clearly established, is, under certain circumstances, positively morbific. Several instances are on record of death occurring on exposure to the exhalations from putrid corpses; and, according to Baron Percy, at an anatomical demonstration in Paris, — decomposition of the subject being far advanced, — the celebrated Fourcroy, after being exposed to the emanations from the decaying body, suffered from a violent eruptive fever; that one of the physicians died in three days, in consequence of breathing the tainted air; and that two others remained for a long time in a debilitated condition, from which one never entirely recovered.

Dr. Good states, that, in opening some of the burial-places of France, the effluvium strikes so forcibly upon the grave-digger as to throw him into a state of asphyxia, if close at hand; and, if at a little distance, to oppress him with vertigo, fainting, nausea, loss of appetite, and tremors, for several hours; while numbers of those who live in the neighborhood of such cemeteries labor under dejected spirits, sallow countenances, and febrile emaciation. Many similar relations might be added, were it necessary; and, although it would be perhaps difficult to prove that exposure to animal decomposition would invariably affect health in a directly perceptible manner, yet that effluvia from human bodies in a state of decay do, in many individuals and under many conditions, act most injuriously, tending to excite nervous and putrid disorders, destroying health and life, is an assertion which no one probably will undertake to refute. Magendie has expressed his decided conviction, that the miasm arising from church-yards, and which is often perceptible to the olfactory sense of the inhabitants of cities, is a fruitful source of disease, decrepitude, and death; even though much diluted by the atmosphere, and spread over a large extent of country.

The existence of a dense crowd of living beings, men, dogs, and horses, confined within the narrow limits of a city, is sufficient to vitiate the air, and render it unfavorable to health, without the presence of the dead. Notwithstanding the best-regulated sanitary measures, even if constantly carried on with the commendable energy which characterized the proceedings of our city authorities in view of the recent pestilence; notwithstanding the multiplication of "breathing holes," those "lungs of a metropolis" to which the half-stifled citizen may resort when he can "spare time" to inhale the "pure air of heaven," there will necessarily exist many sources of impurity, much that breeds disease, exclusive of the contamination of sepulchres. The mortality of a city is much greater than that of the country. The favorable change frequently effected by a removal from the former to the latter, particularly in diseases connected with the respiratory organs, is strikingly indicative of the comparative insalubrity of a town-residence. And not to the invalid alone is the change beneficial. All have experienced, on passing into the open country, the invigorating, exhilarating influence of pure air, — that blessed, health-sustaining agent of which men are so wilfully deprived when "jamming themselves" between the brick walls of a narrow and crowded city, "the hospital of the living, and the tomb of the dead."

Allusion has been made to moisture in the atmosphere as apparently tending to promote the spread of malarious diseases. The exciting poison is unquestionably exhaled from the earth, whatever may be the nature of the exhalations; but it is evident that moisture enters largely into the circumstances which favor the extension and concentration of the miasm. In general, the diseases which are evidently produced by the poisonous emanations from the soil prevail in marshy districts, where, through the influence of solar heat, evaporation loads the air with moisture. It is true that, in dry, elevated situations, the same diseases have been known to exist; a fact attempted to be explained on the presumption that the miasma, which, by reason of its greater specific gravity, would remain near the surface of the earth, is raised by the lighter ascending vapor to a higher and dryer locality. Independently of its presumed agency in the transmission of poisonous properties, atmospheric moisture is more unfavorable to health than the opposite condition, dryness. Sir Jas. Clarke asserts, that "humidity, of all the physical qualities of the air, is the most injurious to human life." He adds, that "particular attention should be paid, in selecting situations for building, to the circumstances which are calculated to obviate humidity either in the soil or atmosphere, in every climate. Thick and lofty trees, close to a house, tend to maintain the air in a state of humidity, by preventing its free circulation, and by obstructing the free admission of the sun's rays. Houses in confined, shady situations, with damp courts or gardens, or standing water close to them, are unhealthy in every climate and season, but especially in a country subject to intermitting fevers, and during summer and autumn."

In travelling from Civita Vecchia to Rome, over a portion of the Pontine Marshes, the sad consequences of inhaling air rendered impure by earthy exhalations are strikingly visible upon the health of the unfortunate inhabitants there met with. Vegetating slowly and laboriously like sickly plants, struggling vainly against the deadly influence of the malaria, with complexions sallow and corpse-like, eyes sunken and lustreless, limbs "doughy" and dropsical, imbecile in mind and body, they wander gloomily about, drinking in, with every breath, the poison which early consumes them.

At no period of life are the deleterious consequences of confinement in impure air more perceptible than during infancy and childhood. "Pale countenances, weak eyes, general relaxation of the body, an accumulation of all the inconveniences and sufferings of childhood, at length consumption, and early dissolution of life, are the natural and frequent consequences of such confinement. The daily enjoyment of fresh air contributes greatly to the health and sprightliness of children, and is one of the most efficient preventives against that delicate and sickly condition which is so frequently witnessed in those who are almost constantly confined and pampered in nurseries." — (*Eberle.*) "Pure, uncontaminated air is, indeed, most grateful to the feelings of children. After having been carried out but a few times, they evince, even at a very early age, a strong desire to return to the open air. When they can scarcely crawl, they instinctively advance towards that part of the room from which they have a prospect of escaping." — (*Struve.*)

CHAPTER IV.

ON EXERCISE.

Health cannot be sustained without exercise. The due development of the muscles into elastic firmness; the energetic action of the digestive apparatus; the easy, unobstructed circulation of the blood; healthy absorption, secretion, and nutrition, are all dependent upon a proper degree of bodily exertion. There is no hygienic agent of more consequence, none which requires such incessant urging by the medical attendant upon patients invalided through indolence, and no curative influence more thoroughly, systematically neglected, than exercise. With muscles torpid from want of action, nerves unstrung, digestion painful, mind enfeebled, the snail-imitating immortal, wearied with doing nothing, "ennuyed" by the merest trifle, fancies that he requires medicine; and, when told that activity is the grand restorative, resorts to the favorite easy-chair, and smiles incredulously; or, if prevailed upon to make an effort, crawls lazily through a few streets, and returns to lie down, as though completely exhausted. There are hundreds in this melancholy condition; men and women dying from inaction, "stagnating like sluggish pools;" while the world is full of objects demanding human interest and human energy.

The desire for muscular action is exhibited in the earliest years of man. It is a powerful instinct of animal nature. There is an involuntary tendency in the young to move energetically and freely; and they would be gamboling most of the time, were not their little frames "cribbed, coffined, and confined" on the hard benches of a hot school-room, or compelled by their fond parents to keep quiet at home. Physical activity is a necessity with all animate things; it is a law universal throughout creation, that health and subsistence are to be gained by exertion, "by the sweat of the brow." Adam was not born in a rocking chair, before a coal fire, and requested to sit still and make himself comfortable. He was obliged to move after means of subsistence, to dig for roots, to climb for fruit, or to chase the animals for a meal; and it would be better for all his descendants, morally and physically, were they compelled to do the same.

By exercise, an invigorating impulse is communicated, through the accelerated circulation, to every portion of the living frame. Respiration is more full and free; the cutaneous vessels are stimulated; the appetite increased; the muscular and nervous systems strengthened; secretory action promoted; obstructions prevented; the spirits enlivened; every function of the body and every faculty of the mind animated with natural, healthful energy. It is cruel, in view of these advantages, to impose restraint upon the motions of childhood. It is a sad self-infliction for the adult to deprive himself of such beneficial results. It would be folly to make a fixture of a machine adapted for locomotion, allowing it to rust and be ruined in unprofitable inaction. How much greater is the folly when that machine is a living, breathing, naturally-restless thing, every fibre gifted with full powers of action and endurance, with a wonderful arrangement of moving forces, and a "spark of divinity" enclosed that will live for ever, dimmed and nearly extinguished by the unhealthy, unnatural stillness of its enveloping material, upon whose movements, in no small degree, its brightness depends!

Sedentary occupations, unless regular intervals are allotted for exercise, induce a condition the very reverse of health. Mechanics of a certain class are liable to diseases of which the active man knows nothing. Artists, gilders, watchmakers, tailors, and others of like occupation, are subject to peculiar bodily derangements. Congestion to the lungs and abdomen, gastric difficulties, nervous headaches, irritability and weakness of body and mind, which render the man a burden to himself and an annoyance to those around him, result from long-continued and close confinement to such employments. Regular, methodical exercise, which would counteract the evil effects of such a life, because it does not appear directly "profitable," is neglected; and thus too many needlessly fall victims to complaints which embitter their whole existence. When the business demands much mental application, when intense study is added to want of exercise, the consequences are still more disastrous. Instances of longevity are extremely rare among those who devote their hours to incessant application. Constitutions endowed by nature with unusual power "break down" in the very "spring-time of life," without relaxation. Men of rugged frames and nerves of iron, who might have fitted themselves almost to cope with the lion in his strength, and to match the antelope in agility, become, in a few brief years, puny and helpless, and early fall a resistless prey to that mortal enemy of the studious man, — inactivity. How widely different is the physical training of the civilized citizen and the savage! The daily labor of the former frequently consists in merely varying the position of his lower extremities by forcing a four-legged chair to become a biped, and by raising his heels above the level of his head. The savage, on the contrary, is in constant activity. His limbs are supple, springy, and powerful. His pedestrian excursions are somewhat more extensive than the five minutes' travel of a sickly student; for they are forty or fifty miles in length; and when he sits or lies down, it is for the purpose of resting. After resting, he is refreshed, and with renewed vigor, and in the wild exhilaration of high health, bounds forth, with a shout, into the free air to procure his food.

The institution of the Olympic games by Lycurgus, after the Trojan war, tended more than any other of his wise regulations to prevent the ancient Greeks from becoming luxurious and effeminate. The most important of these games were wrestling, boxing, quoit-pitching, foot and horse-racing; and to excel in such exercises, which were conducted with a view to the development of bodily and mental strength, was an honor to which all aspired, — a victory which inflamed their ambition more even than the acquisition of military glory. An indolent Greek was, in those days, an object of scorn and contempt. The Romans encouraged their youth to exercise in the Gymnasiums, as the surest method of forming a nation of strong and brave soldiers; and, during the middle ages, when warlike operations were going on throughout the continent of Europe, when physical energy and activity were of the highest value on the field of battle, manly sports were engaged in with intense ardor by all classes of people, as the principal means of bestowing health and strength. And, in England, exercises in the open air were regarded as of such consequence, in the formation of manliness of person and character, that royal proclamations and parliamentary acts were repeatedly promulgated for their promotion and regulation.

The youth of the present age, inheriting a predisposition to chronic diseases, the ultimate effect, perhaps, of indolent habits contracted by the parents, are reared like hot-house plants, that the "wind of heaven may not visit them too roughly," instead of being subjected to means which forward organic development, and counterbalance a scrofulous or consumptive tendency. The germ of disease is fostered with extraordinary care, until it attains an exuberance of growth which defies all remedial measures; and, in the morning of life, a premature grave is opened for the burial of the poor victim to persevering mismanagement. At variance with every known physical law, in contradiction to all that is reasonable and self-evident, is the too prevalent notion that weakly children should be at rest. Withholding from the feverish sufferer the only refrigerating diluent (cold water) which nature is urgently demanding; shutting out from the suffocating invalid the fresh air for which he gasps; binding down the quivering muscle already debilitated by unnatural inaction, are absurdities analogous in character, and practices abhorrent to every pathological and physiological principle.

With regard to the various modes of exercise, *walking* is generally the most serviceable to health, as it is the most simple and convenient. A more equal distribution of motion is imparted to the muscular apparatus; a more unconstrained position is assumed in this quiet mode of progression than in any other. It is an exercise in which the rich and the poor can, at all times, indulge; and for the neglect of which no possible excuse, by the sound-limbed, can be offered. By walking is not meant the lazy dragging of one foot after the other across a street, or from the dwelling-house to the shop or office; but a brisk, vigorous, resolute propulsion of the body far out into the pure air of the country, where the eye can rest upon objects that are not wholly artificial, the ear listen to music more exhilarating than the noise of cart-wheels and voices of charcoal vendors, and the soul refreshed by being elevated "through nature up to nature's God." A man may hurry through the crowded streets of a city, dodging at every step to avoid violent contact with posts, animate and inanimate, until he is fatigued and irritated; a woman may perform her domestic duties with considerable agility, running up and down staircases until she is "out of breath," and beguile herself with the idea that such spasmodic movements are all that health requires. But much of the benefit of exercise is lost, unless accompanied by the inspiration of fresh air. The circulation of the blood is accelerated by muscular exertion, and the motion of the lungs is thereby increased; but, for the healthy oxygenation of the augmented flow of blood, pure air is positively needed; and the more rapid the respiration, the more necessity exists for the inhalation of pure air. The women of England and Scotland, in general, walk twelve to fifteen miles daily. It becomes a pleasurable excitement, as well as a salutary recreation; and the advantages are visible in the cheerful expression of countenance, the long-retained fresh bloom of youth, and the well-developed frame. We allude not to the idle, pampered aristocracy, nor to the opposite extreme of society; but to the middle classes, who are interested in the cultivation of their health, and have sense enough to appreciate its value. How melancholy is the contrast of these happy results with the condition of our own countrywomen; who, with unhealthy looking, emaciated faces and figures, grown prematurely aged by confinement in the impure air of their dwellings, venture out only in perfectly pleasant weather, and are then "tired almost to death," after the walk of a mile or two!

Dancing is an exercise frequently referred to by its votaries as greatly conducive to health. It would be so, doubtless, for it is a movement well adapted to bring the muscles into united action, were the climate such as to admit of its practice in the open air; but when conducted, as it necessarily is with us, in heated ball-rooms, at midnight, in thin dresses, vitiated air, and with the liability of exposure to extreme changes of temperature, it cannot be recommended when attended by such circumstances, as an exercise promotive of health. The ball-room, in truth, too often proves the introduction to a sad scene of suffering, terminated only by death.

Riding on horseback is rather a passive sort of exercise, but is beneficial as well as agreeable, and better adapted than any other for those who suffer from a torpid condition of the gastric and hepatic functions. Unless, however, the motion of the animal is easy, or the rider well taught, strong muscular contraction is required to preserve an equipoise; and the feeble and delicate system is subjected to efforts which may prove too violent. The favorable consequences are very decided with those who complain of indigestion, and the endless variety of anomalous derangements which have no fixedness, resulting from sedentary occupations. It has been highly recommended by some for the consumptive; but the benefits which appear to have arisen may have been more from the change of air and scene than from any peculiar influence of the exercise itself. Opinions relative to its suitableness are singularly contradictory. Sydenham affirms that none of the so-called specifics, which are used with such confidence for their appropriate diseases, are more effectual than saddle exercise in "phthisis." Stoll, on the contrary, says that, if a consumptive patient mount his horse, he will ride straight to the banks of the Styx. Dr. Parrish recommends daily and long-continued riding on horseback as the best mode of exercise, even when pulmonary consumption is present. A highly esteemed friend, the late Dr. Worcester, of Cincinnati, stated to the writer, that, while laboring under unequivocal symptoms of tubercular phthisis, he turned his horse's head westward, and rode as on a "steeple-chase," more than one thousand miles, through swamps and over fences, through rivers and over mountains, in one almost undeviating line; and, on his return to Cincinnati, his health for a time was completely restored.

The athletic exercises of the gymnasium contribute to the preservation, and, if practised with moderation and judgment, to the restoration of health. It is necessary to observe, however, that muscular exertion, by those who have not gradually accustomed themselves to severe exercise, may be carried to an injurious extent; producing such irregularity of action in all the functions, as to lead to serious organic mischief. The desperate activity which young, ambitious athletæ occasionally force themselves to exhibit, for the admiration of their friends, may occasion aneurism of the arteries and enlargement of the heart, ruptures, lacerations, &c. Whenever powerful efforts are made from the chest as a centre, blood is determined, through the retention of breath, to the head, and congestions are liable to occur therein, as well as ruptures of vessels or transudation of the contained fluid through their coats. There may be intemperance in exercise, as in all other things; and, when it exceeds the bounds of moderation, when carried to the point of exhaustion, injury instead of benefit will result.

As an evidence of the decided effects of judicious gymnastic management, the following case is related by Dr. Rosentein:—

"In Berne, Switzerland, a child, three years old, could scarcely stand upon his legs. At five years, he could walk with the assistance of a leading string; and it was not before he was seven years old that he commenced to walk without aid. He would, however, frequently fall, and could not rise without exertion. At seventeen, his strength was so feeble that his limbs could scarcely bear the weight of the upper part of his body. He felt great weakness in his arms, his shoulders were drawn forward, his breast narrow, his breathing short, and his mental capacities not much developed.

"In 1815, this unfortunate being was sent to the gymnastic school of Mr. Clias, in Berne. Having measured his strength by the pressure of his hands applied to the dynamometer, it was calculated to be equal to that of a child of seven years of age. The powers of traction, ascension, running, were null. In one minute and two seconds, he could scarcely walk the distance of a hundred steps; and when he reached the end of his little journey, he felt exhausted, and was obliged to sit down and rest himself. The weight of fifteen pounds put into his hands made him stagger; and a child of seven years could easily throw him down. Five months later, through gymnastic exercise and a suitable diet, his powers increased to double the sum. He could, by means of his arms, raise himself three inches from the ground, and remain three seconds in that position. He could jump a distance of three feet; run a hundred and sixty-three steps in a minute, carrying along with him, on the shoulders, thirty-five pounds weight. In 1817, in the presence of thousands of spectators, he could climb up a rope twenty feet high, and repeat the same manœuvre on a climbing pole, jump a distance of six feet, and run five hundred steps in two minutes and a half. In 1818, he could walk five miles without the least fatigue. And this same person, who at twenty years of age could scarcely carry himself erect, became, through this healthful exercise, a strong and vigorous man, and could, in combat, put most men at defiance."

Exercise of every description should be commenced *gently*. The transition from dead inactivity to violent exertion may be dangerously precipitate. There is no propensity requiring more restraint than that tendency of "rushing into extremes" with which the North American is so uncomfortably afflicted. Calm but determined perseverance is better adapted for success, in physical as well as moral and religious reformation, than the fierce, restless, quickly exhausted energy of the enthusiast. The sententious axiom, "Be sure you are right, then go ahead," of our eccentric countryman, who appeared vastly desirous of being considered "a horse," does not necessarily imply and need not be accompanied, in its application to practice, by that equally favorite vulgarism, "Go ahead, if you break your neck." "Be moderate in all things" is a scriptural phrase of most important hygienic signification, — a text capable of profitable expatiation, and demanding, in this age of independent thought and action, the especial attention of "Young America."

Exercise should also be taken regularly; in the pure open air, if possible; and never directly after a meal.

CHAPTER V.

ON BATHING.

FOR the establishment and preservation of health, there is no hygienic expedient more easily adopted and more carelessly regarded than bathing; and, for the restoration of health, there is no single therapeutic measure which has been more neglected and more abused. The dislike — the positive repugnance — of the large class of "the unwashed" to the application of water to other portions of the skin than those which are exposed to the air, perhaps results from its prohibition in the clinical practice of former times, — in the obstinate proscription by physicians of this invigorating refrigerant, as a very hazardous external resort during sickness. The opposite absurdity of applying cold water to the body in profusion and indiscriminately, — as well to the sensitive, delicate infant as to the feeble, aged adult, — at all times and seasons, and under all conditions, may be attributed to the enthusiastic hydropathist. Between the two extremes, as in all things else, there is a "golden mean," by which the rational and consistent may abide.

The skin exercises a very important function in the animal economy. By its secretory vessels, which are composed of the extremities of the cutaneous arteries, a vapor is continually exhaled from the surface, in an imperceptible form usually, but made visible when the vessels are stimulated by external or internal heat, or by powerful mental emotion. This watery vapor is a secretion — like all other secretions — furnished from the blood, and health is dependent upon its uninterrupted exhalation. By insensible perspiration, the blood is freed from superfluous matter, consisting of water, acetic and carbonic acid, muriate of soda and potash, earthy phosphate, and oxide of iron. By sensible perspiration, especially when produced by active therapeutic measures, the miasmata which have originated disease, as well as medicines which have been taken in a crude state, and have consequently promoted or as is probable caused disease, are expelled through the pores of the skin. As any obstruction to the free passage of this secretion, through its innumerable outlets upon the surface of the body, must of necessity interrupt in a measure the secreting process, it is evidently a point of considerable consequence to remove, or if possible prevent, such obstructions. Now, these obstructions are constantly liable to occur from the presence of particles of dust or of clothing, or from the perspiration itself, the saline particles of which remain in contact with the skin after the aqueous portion has evaporated; and washing the skin frequently with water is the most efficient means which can be taken to prevent the accumulation of such obstructing causes.

During the process of respiration, vapor is exhaled from the lungs, and the quantity is increased if by any means cutaneous perspiration is obstructed. The deficiency must thus be made up by the lungs, if the free exercise of the functions of the skin is interfered with. Should the latter be the case, respiration must be more than commonly laborious; and this over-exertion of the lungs unavoidably tends to debility, and induces consumption, and other diseases of the chest. To offer every facility, therefore, for the promotion of free, unobstructed transpiration, is to adopt a precautionary measure against the occurrence of pulmonary disease, which, as is too well known, needs in our climate but very little encouragement. The escape of the evaporable portion of the perspiration may be promoted by the use of light and porous material worn next the skin, and, on the contrary, prevented by clothing impermeable to air and moisture. But the impurities which do not evaporate, and which are ever accumulating, cannot be removed except by ablution with water; and such ablution should be performed daily.

Bathing in *cold water* is practised much more generally now than at any former period. That it is an agent of vast importance in the preservation of health is undeniable. It acts favorably, not only by cleansing the skin from impurities, but, by its secondary effect, increasing the action of the cutaneous vessels, strengthening the nervous system, promoting vigorous circulation, and rendering the body more capable of enduring with impunity the rapid alternations of atmospheric temperature. The immediate effect of its application to the healthy frame is depressing. The action of the capillaries, or perspiratory organs, that of the nervous and vascular systems, and even of the mental, are diminished. When re-action takes place, indicated by a sensation of warmth, all the animal functions are carried on with renewed energy, and its happy influence is exhibited in the re-animation and increased capability of both the physical and mental powers. This re-action is the measure of advantage derived. If occurring early, and in a marked manner, the application of cold has proved beneficial. If, on the contrary, the primary action continues long, the sensation of chilliness not being followed by that of warmth, but accompanied by debility and exhaustion, the bathing is of doubtful advantage, or rather of decided injury. It is evident, that, where re-action does not take place, — where there is a deficiency of vital activity, from whatever cause arising, — the influence which adds to the previous depression of the powers of life, and is prolonged in its action, must be an unfavorable one.

Re-action does not readily occur in the debilitated and delicate, nor in infancy or old age, when the vital functions are feebly executed. It may be favored, however, when delayed, by friction with some coarse material. Friction, with or without bathing, it should be observed, is an eligible substitute for exercise, when the latter cannot be conveniently taken. Although it is not attended with all the advantages derived from exercise in the open air, it nevertheless invigorates the muscular fibre, through sympathy with the cutaneous vessels, and increases the energy of the whole system.

The external use of cold water has been recommended by some as safe in all seasons, for all ages, and in all conditions. Those who practise indiscriminately upon such irrational advice will be led into great error. It is certainly not beneficial to very young children, as an extreme susceptibility to cold exists during the period of infancy, and the system resists with difficulty the influence of any sudden change. The consequence of a powerful impression of this kind to the sensitive membrane, enclosing the whole delicate mechanism of young life, is a rapid repulsion of blood from the entire surface upon the vital organs, and an irritation, by sympathetic action, of the internal mucous membranes, thereby causing convulsions, croup, bowel complaints, &c. This conclusion has not been admitted as legitimate by many; but it is, nevertheless, one which will demand

7

more than a simple denial to controvert. The temperature of water ought to be *gradually* reduced when applied to infants, as well as when used by the feeble and aged. It should be constantly modified to suit particular cases, as well when adopted for the prevention as for the cure of disease.

To the hydropathic method of treatment, no reference need here be made, excepting to observe, that, whatever may have been its advantages in certain disorders, as a *system* of cure it appears wholly incomplete. That it has proved effectual in many complaints, that the "wet sheet," for example, has been productive of very great advantage in certain stages of fever, is certain; but it is also as certain, that the practice, in any of its forms, is neither applicable to all diseases, nor to be safely administered to all persons, under all circumstances. As an occasional auxiliary to the internal action of medicines prepared according to the direction of Hahnemann, who originated the only method of practice worthy of being called a system, it finds its true place in therapeutics.

The especial curative power of cold applications, made use of to a partial extent, when the skin is preternaturally hot and dry, consists in its reducing the temperature of the surface with which they come into contact. The diminution of action thus locally caused is communicated by sympathy to every portion of the cutaneous system of vessels, modifying the morbid heat throughout the body. By this force and extent of sympathy it is that the disposition to inflammation of throat and lungs may be counteracted by the frequent application of cold water to the feet; the temperature of the water being gradually reduced, when there is reason to apprehend a deficient re-action. It should here be added, that, always with the restriction above named, the practice of frequently bathing the feet in cold water lessens the susceptibility to those sudden variations of temperature to which these useful members are constantly subjected during winter. The habit of "toasting" them several hours before a hot fire, and directly afterward rushing out upon the snow-covered sidewalk, is one much more common than prudent; and some fortifying process is absolutely necessary. The epitaph, "Died of thin shoes," would not be such a generally applicable inscription over the grave of the young and beautiful, were the feet more frequently prepared against exposure by the invigorating influence of a daily cold bath.

The *warm bath*, or that which exceeds in temperature the natural warmth of the body, is far more conducive to disease than to health. By its use, the excitability of the system is greatly increased, the circulation accelerated, the respiration embarrassed, the tendency to plethora developed; and the perspiration induced terminates in a state of languor and exhaustion. When the water used is 10 or 15 degrees lower than the temperature of the body, which is about 96 degrees of Fahrenheit, its operation in some cases is positively beneficial; for it acts as an admirable sedative in those conditions of irritability consequent upon fatigue or great excitement, and it is, above all, advantageous, as preparatory to the more tonic influence of the actual cold bath, for the feeble and delicate.

The same observations will apply to the shower bath, — to its consequences as regards temperature; viz. that the depression following its application, when cold water is employed, is too great in cases where re-action is with difficulty accomplished; that, under such conditions, tepid water should be used. It is the most advisable mode, however, of applying water when there exists a predisposition to certain cerebral affections.

The most convenient mode of ablution is that which consists in the use of a wet sponge or towel, the surface being rubbed briskly with a dry cloth directly after the cold application. A wash-bowl is the most portable and the most ready bathing machine. The habit, once formed, of daily ablution in this manner, graduating the temperature of the water to the bather's sensations, will not only be found the best measure of prevention against those affections incident to our variable climate, but greatly promotive of strength, cheerfulness, and longevity.

The hour selected for bathing is an important point for consideration. While digestion is going on, three hours being the average time for that operation, any strong impulse communicated from without to the circulatory and nervous systems disturbs the process by withdrawing from the digestive organs the vital force which they require. Directly after rising in the morning is the most favorable time in general; but for those who need immediate subsequent exercise to promote a healthy re-action, the third hour after breakfast is the one most suitable. The system is oftener enervated than re-animated by a night's repose, in civilized life, and is unable to endure well much early exercise without sustenance.

Under the head of bathing, one of our best writers on hygiene, Dr. Dunglison, of Philadelphia, alludes in the following terms, which we take the liberty of quoting, to the practice of resorting to watering places for the restoration of health. The remarks are not perhaps directly applicable to the subject of this chapter; but they cannot be more appropriately introduced in any other place. He mentions having, in his work on "General Therapeutics," "animadverted on the evil that must necessarily result in various diseases from the indiscriminate mode in which different mineral waters are drunk at their sources; and to a less degree the evil is experienced when they are employed by those in health; and has there remarked that every intelligent physician, at fashionable watering places, has deplored the ignorance of invalids and their medical advisers, which has doomed many a hopeless case to a most inconvenient pilgrimage; for although the accommodations at such places ought to be adapted expressly for the comfort of the sick, attention appears to be paid rather to the sound, who are able to enjoy the pleasures of the table." He adds that "nothing is more preposterous than the practice almost universally inculcated and followed at different mineral springs, of directing immense quantities of the water to be taken early before breakfast: ten tumblersfull is not an uncommon quantity at Saratoga; and, accordingly, we ought not to be astonished, that so many persons visit these and other mineral springs of the country in the possession of health, and leave them in a state of disease; when, if they had taken the waters in moderation, the tone of their systems might have been materially improved. · It is absurd to prescribe the same formula for all cases, and to load the stomach so much in any case; yet such is the popular custom at most of the watering places.

"If the sojourner at the springs be in good health, let him avoid the waters altogether, or take them sparingly, leaving the other hygienic influences to be fully exerted upon him; but, should he be a valetudinarian, the waters must be had recourse to under appropriate rules, suggested by the nature of the case, and the peculiar mineral impregnation. Few, however, of the searchers after health will believe that the least important hygienic agent is the water; and, were they convinced of this, they might perhaps be less disposed to visit, and pass their time at, the springs, and to reap the other extrinsic advantages to which allusion has been made. The drinking of the waters is an object for undertaking a journey; and, if the journey be undertaken, it may happen that the use of the waters will be found unnecessary, if not injurious."

CHAPTER VI.

ON CLOTHING.

A FEW observations in relation to the covering necessary to protect the body from the influence of cold will not be out of place here. Many complaints resulting in death may be directly traced to carelessness with regard to dress. That material which is the worst conductor of caloric is the best protection against external heat or cold; for animal heat which would otherwise be dissipated is thus retained, and atmospheric heat also prevented from acting upon the surface of the body. Flannel is the article of clothing which best answers this condition, and it may be worn under or over linen. It has been objected to as increasing the susceptibility to external impressions; but the objection applies to many varieties of clothing. Undoubtedly it would be better were the surface rendered, in a great measure, insensible to cold by the early practice of frequent bathing, commenced, as has been already remarked, by the use of tepid water, and gradually reduced, in temperature, to the freezing point.

When the system has thus become habituated to the sudden abstraction of heat, the vicissitudes of climate may be endured with comparative impunity, even if no addition is made to the linen or cotton usually worn in summer next the skin. But where this preservative habit is not in force; where, from negligence or necessity, a debilitated condition prevails, — an incapacity of re-acting against agencies to which the body must be exposed, — the protection afforded by flannel is greater than from any other material. Independently of its being a bad conductor of caloric, it acts advantageously by stimulating in a degree the cutaneous vessels, and by absorbing, in consequence of its loose texture, much of the impurities thrown out by perspiration, which would otherwise, especially if bathing were not frequently practised, accumulate upon the skin. It is believed also that the poisonous exhalations from the earth, in certain localities, are rendered less injurious to health by the use of flannel. Travellers over the marshes in the vicinity of Rome are recommended to wear it, as one of the chief preservatives against the noxious action of malaria.

It is not to be denied, that much mischief results from the wearing of woollen or any other fabric which induces perspiration. Sensible perspiration, in a healthy person, should be produced by no other means than exercise. An excess of covering, as well during the day as the night, is relaxing and debilitating. The quantity promotive of comfort, one's own sensations being the guide, is the only rule of safety.

Much attention ought to be given to the clothing of infants. At this period of life, the power of generating heat is less than at any other time. The great mortality in infancy is justly attributed to a deficiency of clothing, in connection with vitiated air and improper diet. In some counties of France, the birth of every child must be registered by the mayor of the district, and the personal presence of the infant is required. It happens, that, where this regulation exists, more than common inattention is paid to the clothing of these little creatures, and it has been found that a great number perish in consequence of this exposure; while the deaths are much more numerous in the cold than in warm seasons; and a much larger proportion occurs among those who are brought from a distance, than among those in the neighborhood of the Registry Office.

As the quantity of clothing should be regulated by the sensations of comfort, it is equally important that those sensations should be consulted with reference to the tightness of the dress. No compression ought to be permitted; no hindrance to the free and easy movement of the muscles, or to the full expansion of the lungs. It was one of the most foolish decrees of that foolish goddess, Fashion, that her votaries should be forced to respire in a laborious manner;

should suffer from constriction of the thoracic and abdominal portions of the frame, or be exposed to apoplexy by the pressure of a tight cravat upon the vessels of the neck. It would be perhaps superfluous to expatiate here upon the folly of compressing the waist by tight lacing. If this error is persisted in at the present day, it cannot be from ignorance of its disastrous consequences, since the practice has been stigmatized in every publication issued on physiology, and in every lecture delivered on the laws of health, since the commencement of the nineteenth century. No part of the healthy human body, from the crown of the head to the sole of the feet, will admit of compression without injury, unless it be temporarily adopted with a view to the immediate support of some debilitated internal organ. Uneasiness and constraint, experienced even in the feet, frequently bring on sympathetic affections of a serious nature in the chest and head; and an impeded circulation, by local pressure anywhere, will ultimately result in a diminution of strength and disturbance of health.

In concluding these remarks on clothing, it may not be improper to advert to the covering which Providence has provided for man, and of which he sees fit, at the sacrifice of a vast amount of time and comfort, to deprive himself. Necessarily more exposed to atmospheric influences, in his capacity of purveyor for a household, than the "softer sex," he has been furnished with a protection not only for the neck behind, but also for the neck in front, and a large portion of the face. The beard which defends the throat, — the whiskers and moustache which are probably designed for a similar purpose with regard to the teeth, — the eyebrows, which guard, to a certain extent, the eye, — are all equally useful. This hair was intended to answer some valuable end as an integument, or it would not have been permitted to grow; and the caprice of fashion is in no particular more obviously absurd, than when leading man to flourish a dangerously sharp instrument about his nose, ears, and throat, daily, from the age of maturity until death, in order to cut down that which is of no possible use to any one, after being removed. If it is equally useless before its removal, it certainly proves a strange and solitary exception to that beautiful law of design, — the adaptation of means to an end, — which prevails throughout nature.

CHAPTER VII.

ON SLEEP.

Among the necessary means of renovating the vital energies, and recruiting the nervous system, is that of sleep; a condition in which there is a suspension of the voluntary activity that would soon exhaust, if uninterrupted, the powers of life. The functions of nutrition continue in operation; all muscular motion not dependent on volition goes on, though with retarded action; while the senses are closed to external impressions, and the crowd of earth-born influences which "war against the soul" is lost to cognizance. If this cessation of muscular and mental activity does not take place, if unceasing application or artificial stimulants prolong the interval of wakefulness beyond a certain point, nervous action is unhealthy, and the whole physical system becomes enfeebled and diseased. The privation of sleep, like that of food and drink, is the withholding a necessity which nature imperatively demands. Regularity in the use of the three necessaries of life is important; and indulgence in one as in the other, beyond the actual requirements of the system, tends to the deterioration of health.

The re-instatement of nervous energy, to be effected by repose, must be disturbed in its progress through any cause which interrupts sleep. The more tranquil the condition, the more salutary will be its effects. For the promotion of quiet, refreshing sleep, digestion, which is executed with less facility in this state, should not be excited by a full supper before retiring to rest. Dreams of an unpleasant nature are frequently the consequence of an overloaded stomach; and most people have experienced the nervous exhaustion resulting from frightful impressions upon the mind, when sleep has deprived it of the guidance of judgment.

A hard, unyielding surface is no more conducive to healthy repose than the soft mass of feathers upon or in which many persons luxuriate. The best bed is the common hair mattress; neither too hard to be uncomfortable, nor so yielding as to induce restlessness. The covering should be thick enough to preserve warmth, without causing perspiration.

Reference has already been made to an obvious source of unhealthiness generally attendant on sleep, viz. the confined air in bed-chambers. It is vain to hope for re-invigoration and refreshment from a night's rest, however favorable may be all other attendant circumstances, if the blood is to be poisoned, through the medium of the lungs, by air, impure perhaps at first, and inhaled over and over again for several consecutive hours. Every window and door in a bedroom ought to be opened to their utmost capacity, in the morning if at no other time, and all the bed-clothing well and thoroughly aired, if either health or cleanliness is to be consulted.

Another important consideration is the amount of time passed in sleep. During this period, the circulation is of course going on, and transpiration, at the whole surface of the body, of the waste material, is not only undiminished, but rather increased; while neither food nor exercise furnishes counter-balancing supplies to the system. If this state of things is continued beyond the requisite time for the restoration of nervous energy, the consequence must inevitably be a gradual diminution of vital force, resulting ultimately in the complete prostration of the bodily and mental faculties. In early life, sleep is more necessary than at a maturer age, when the functions of the nervous system are less energetic. Eight hours of the twenty-four are sufficient for any adult who is in health, and much more than has been indulged in by many eminent men distinguished for activity, of whose domestic habits history has informed us. Napoleon spent but four hours in sleep, during the most active portion of a life remarkable for exhibitions of mental and physical energy. Many have been contented with even less. Instances of this kind, however, should be excepted as peculiar; for there are but few constitutions that do not require longer repose. "Seven hours for a man, eight hours for a woman, and nine hours for a fool," is an old saying in reference to the proper duration of sleep, the authority for which it would not be worth while to give, even if it were known. The time allotted to the man is doubtless suitable, but it is not physiologically true that women require more sleep than men: as to the fool, it matters but little how long he *does* sleep; and it is fair to presume that none of that class would be very much interested in hygienic measures of any description.

The time of sleep should be so regulated as to admit of *early rising*. Sir John Sinclair, who had closely investigated the causes of longevity, states, in his work upon that subject, that he had never heard or read of a single case of great longevity where the individual was not an early riser. He adds, that long life has been sometimes attained when some one of all the other laws of health had been violated; but he had never known a solitary instance where the constitution had long withstood that undermining, consequent on protracting the hours of repose beyond the wants of the system.

People in fashionable society, to which with bitter irony the term "good" is applied, turn night into day, and waste the precious morning hours in sleep, depriving themselves of the inspiriting influence which early sunlight produces on all the animated creation. The laws of the outward world and the laws of health are alike opposed to this most unnatural practice.

CHAPTER VIII.

ON OCCUPATIONS.

THE deprivation of a suitable amount of air and exercise, to which attention has been already directed, — exhausting bodily labor, the inhalation of volatilized substances, metallic particles or deleterious gases, exposure to extreme variations of temperature, excessive mental application or anxiety,—are circumstances attendant on certain human avocations, which render them to a very considerable extent unhealthy. Vital action may go on, apparently undiminished, for years, under influences the most adverse; and, by the wonderful capacity which the human economy possesses of becoming accustomed to such influences, the injury produced may seem so slight as to be, for a time, overlooked. Yet the effects accumulate; the progress, though slow, is downward; by a gradual diminution of vital force that point is certainly reached, and not far distant, when the constitution sinks irremediably, and the primary and constantly acting cause then stands out, in an hour too late to retrieve the error, a prominent feature of the past.

The unfavorable circumstances above named are not necessarily attendant on the occupations to be mentioned; for, if no means of counteraction could be made available, it would be useless to allude to them in a work of this kind. It is not possible to avoid entirely such causes, but their consequences may be greatly mitigated.

There is no doubt that the occupations which allow of the free use of fresh air and muscular exercise are those most conducive to health and longevity. The following results, in reference to different pursuits as favoring length of life, were published at Berlin, in 1834. To what extent the researches were conducted we are not informed; but the general correctness of the observations were confirmed shortly after by statistics furnished in the "Report on the Sanitary Condition of the Population of Great Britain."

Of	100	Clergymen who had attained the age of 70 and upwards, there were	42
,,	,,	Farmers	40
,,	,,	Commercial men	35
,,	,,	Military men	33
,,	,,	Lawyers	29
,,	,,	Artists	28
,,	,,	Teachers	27
,,	,,	Physicians	24

The above estimate, if too limited for universal

application, is undoubtedly a near approximation to the truth. It will be observed, that the first half of the list, the clergymen excepted, are of those who are necessarily much exposed to the air, and subjected to physical exercise; while the other half are confined principally within doors, the physician excepted, and engaged in quiet, sedentary occupations. It would be somewhat difficult to explain satisfactorily the cause of the vast difference between the length of life of the clergyman and the physician. It may be that the literary labors of the former do not usually demand the constant application that prevents sufficient bodily exercise; and the nature of his study is such as tends, by diffusing cheerfulness, hope, and serenity, to the prolongation of life. But the latter is, from the painful scenes which his avocation compels him to witness, — from the awful responsibility in which he is involved, subject to agonizing mental anxiety, that wears away his health, and is doubtless the chief cause of his comparative early death.

No mention is made, in the foregoing list, of a large portion of our population, — the useful mechanics. There is no reason for believing that their lives are shortened by their occupation, unless that occupation is such as to confine them to a constrained position, or to force them to inhale irritating substances. In the former class may be included shoemakers, tailors, and other like workmen; and in the latter, coppersmiths, plumbers, operative chemists, &c. With regard to the former, much may be accomplished in neutralizing the bad effects of a bent position of the body, by assuming an upright posture as frequently as possible; by taking care to exercise the muscles in the hours of relaxation, which are cramped during the hours of labor. The right angle, formed by the limbs and trunk, which certain occupations oblige men to assume, need not be retained in walking. In an inclined position, a human being must not only propel himself forward, but must, at the same time, resist the power of gravitation. As to those who work upon metals, the impalpable impurities which arise may be in part removed by proper ventilation; and as much that is floating in the air may be absorbed through the skin, particularly particles of lead, and the volatile matter to which druggists and chemists are exposed, it would be proper for all of this class to change their garments frequently, to bathe often, and to remove every particle that may be absorbed, and also that which may enter the system with the food.

The abbreviation of life from intellectual employment has been questioned, since numerous instances of great longevity have occurred among those who have passed their whole lives in deep study; and the cases of impaired health and of early death in such pursuits have been attributed rather to the collateral circumstances, as irregularity of diet, exercise, sleep, &c. than to the direct effect of cerebral disturbance. Dr. Dunglison, from whose admirable work on Hygiene we have already quoted, — after referring to the assertions of Dr. Madden, that literary life frequently terminates in palsy or apoplexy; Petrarch, Linnæus, Copernicus, Lord Clarendon, Rousseau, Marmontel, Richardson, Steele, Phillips, Johnson, Harvey, Wollaston, Porson, and Reid being enumerated as "martyrs to literary glory," — states that the individuals alluded to were not all remarkable for severe application; that they did not all die of apoplexy or palsy; that most of them attained a good old age; and that the habits of some were such as would destroy any person not possessing a constitution of iron. In contradiction to the opinion of James Johnson, which was that a high range of health is incompatible with the most vigorous exertion of the mind, and that this last both requires and induces a standard of health somewhat below par, instancing Virgil, Horace, Voltaire, and Pope in support of the latter assertion, he (Dr. Dunglison) adds, that "an impaired condition of the bodily functions was doubtless present in the cases referred to; and it has existed, and does exist, in numerous others. But these are only coincidences, affording examples of high intellectual attainments and productions, in spite of the bodily infirmities under which those distinguished individuals labored, but by no means showing that they were the consequence of such infirmities. Nothing, indeed, would seem to be clearer than that full intellectual development requires that the different corporeal functions should be faithfully and regularly executed. It is impossible for the mind to aspire to lofty conceptions, or for the various intellectual faculties to be fully accomplished, unless the body is devoid of suffering. Whatever distracts the mind from its own operations enfeebles the results; and nothing does this more effectually and unpropitiously, than suffering of any kind. Every one must have felt the difficulty of bending the intellectual powers on any important topic, when the stomach has been deranged simply by over-distension, and, still more, when food difficult of digestion has been taken; and how much more must this be the case, under the continued pressure of functional or organic disease! It can be easily conceived, however, that, although sickness may interfere with the vigorous exercise of the higher faculties, it may yet be the occasion of greater production than a state of health. Disease or infirm health necessarily confines the invalid, and hence incites to intellectual exercise, for the purpose of dispelling the ennui which such a condition induces; and thus the *production* may be greater, although the *capabilities* may be less."

It must be admitted, however, that, if the limited statistics hitherto furnished on this subject can serve as a reliable measure of comparison in general, those persons engaged in mental avocations are shorter-lived than those whose pursuits are such as to require bodily labor merely. The sedentary habits of the former will no doubt answer as a partial explanation of this difference: still it is reasonable to conclude, that the constant exercise of an organ, upon whose unexcited regularity of action the normal condition of the nervous system is greatly dependent; the unnatural distension of the cerebral vessels by the afflux of blood induced by such exercise; the abstraction of vital energy from other organs to serve the purpose of the over-tasked brain, — must be productive of injurious consequences to health, irrespective of all other unfavorable circumstances. Such, doubtless, is the *tendency* in every case; and, if exhausted, disordered physical functions enervate the mental faculties, the latter, urged to continued exertion, will also affect the physical functions in proportion to the nervous impressibility, and predispose, if not produce, actual bodily derangement.

The process of thought and of digestion cannot well be prosecuted together, for the reason that a greater amount of the vital energy before alluded to is required, both by the stomach and the brain, for the proper performance of their functions. On this account, the application of the same rule that should be enforced in relation to bodily exertion is advisable, viz. that much mental exercise should not be undertaken directly after a meal. And as, in bodily exercise, the muscles may, by systematic, well-regulated training, be made capable of accomplishing much more than they otherwise would be able to do; so may the mind, by discipline in a similar gradual manner, be fitted to undergo an astonishing amount of labor, at comparatively small cost to vitality. Sir Walter Scott, whose writings in vigor of thought and amount of material have rarely been equalled, effectually disciplined his mental capacities, and economized his time; regulating study and recreation so judiciously, that he preserved a high degree of health, and enlivened the social circle, while he was astonishing the world with the powerful productions of his intellect. But, when a refined sense of honor drove him to forget himself to relieve his family from pecuniary embarrassment, and his proud spirit urged and goaded its animal attendant beyond its powers of endurance, exhausted nature sank, — and Scott died; his life sacrificed to an ambition far nobler than that of literary distinction.

CHAPTER IX.

ON DRUGS.

In the investigation of agencies which exercise unfavorable influences upon human health, the effects of none exhibit themselves with more marked prominence than do those arising from the inconsiderate use of medicine. Material, which has not a single nutriment-charged particle, not a principle which is not poison, is thrown into the system, habitually, from the first days of infancy to the closing hours of life. With what wonderful pertinacity is the opinion adhered to, which pathology utterly disowns, that disease is a *substance* existing somewhere in the interior of the body, which must be forcibly removed by a powerful expellant, instead of being recognized as a simple aberration from the natural condition of health, a modification of the vital force. "With such erroneous ideas," Hahnemann writes, "of the material origin and essence of disease, it is by no means surprising, that, in all ages, the obscure as well as the distinguished practitioner, together with the inventors of the most sublime theories, should have for their principal aim the separation and expulsion of a supposed morbid material; and that the indication most frequently established was that of dividing this material, rendering it movable, and expelling it in various ways; purifying the blood by the action of herbal decoctions, thus unloading it of acrid matter and impurities which it *never contained;* drawing off the imaginary principle of the disease mechanically, by means of setons, cauteries, permanent blisters; and, above all, by the expulsion of the pecant matter, as they termed it, by aperients; — all so many attempts to remove a hostile material principle which never did and never could have existed. Now, if we admit that which is an established fact, — namely, that, with the exception of those diseases brought on by the introduction of indigestible or hurtful substances into the alimentary canal and other organs, those produced by foreign bodies penetrating the skin, &c. — there does not exist a single disease that can have a material principle for its cause: on the contrary, all of them are solely and always the special result of an actual and dynamic derangement in the state of health. How absurd, then, must be that method of treatment which depends upon the expulsion of this imaginary principle!

"No one will deny, that the degenerate and impure substances which appear in diseases are any thing else than the mere product of disease itself, which the system can get rid of in a forcible manner, frequently too forcible, without the aid of expellants; and that they are reproduced so long as the disease continues. These substances often appear to the true physician in the shape of morbid symptoms, and aid him in discovering the nature and image of the disease, which he afterwards avails himself of in performing a cure by means of homœopathic agents."

Disease being the result of a modification of the vital force by which functional or organic derangements are induced, it is impossible to cure, without correcting this vital alteration; and all agents directed against effects, although sometimes alleviating temporarily, are not only unavailing in the removal of the cause, but are in themselves productive of a new morbid condition. If gastric derangement exists, removal of the contents of the stomach by emetics will not serve the purpose of counteracting the diseased action, of which the local derangement is the consequence. The abstraction of blood cannot affect, in a curative manner, the morbid condition, which is perhaps inducing changes in the character of the fluid itself. The unhealthy state of the absorbents, which allow of the unnatural accumulation of fluid in dropsy, is not remedied by removing the effusion through an artificial aperture. All medicinal action, of whatever nature, when applied to consequences, is wholly misdirected, and almost invariably injurious.

Homœopathy does not act against consequences. It makes a careful collection of every indication manifested to the senses, — all the phenomena which can, in any measure, throw light upon the proximate cause which produces the external manifestations. The primary agent, having operated, it may be, in the far-distant past to bring on present disease; the moral impressions; all previous and existing influences; every thing, in short, which can be collected to fill up the picture, to form an exact portrait of the particular disease under consideration, are regarded as of equal importance in pointing out a remedy. If the cause cannot always be discovered by human intelligence; if the totality of symptoms does not always indicate the hidden derangement; if the nature of the primary alteration may never be known; it will be evident that there is, notwithstanding, much greater probability of successful treatment in this way, than when the whole artillery of evacuants, antiphlogistics, &c. is brought violently to bear upon effects. The combined assault of disease and the doctor upon one poor delicate organ is too often an intolerable and a fatal infliction. The medicinal agent which will reinstate the harmonious operations of nature *quietly*, for it cannot be done otherwise, is the only true remedy; and all endeavors to cure, while the proximate morbid cause is acting, will be fruitless.

Were a faithful picture to be drawn of all the

results which have followed the practice of resorting to large doses of drugs, it would indeed be frightful. "We could present rather a serious tragedy, if we were to collect all the cases of poisoning by huge doses of powerful medicines by the disciples of *this* physician, and of sanguinary homicide by the imitators of *that* bold surgeon, though they may both enjoy high repute." — (*Medical Gazette.*)

Could all the consequences which have resulted from the use of a single medicinal agent, — for example, that destructive mineral, mercury, — be brought together, so as to be comprehended in one view, it would be impossible for the human eye to look upon a scene of greater devastation and horror. "Gentlemen," said Prof. Chapman, in his address to the students of the *Allœopathic* Medical School in Philadelphia, "if you could see, what I almost daily see in my private practice in this city, persons from the South in the very last stages of wretched existence, emaciated to a skeleton, with both tables of the skull almost completely perforated in many places, the nose half gone, with rotten jaws, ulcerated throats, breaths more pestiferous, more intolerable, than poisonous upas, limbs racked with the pains of the Inquisition, minds as imbecile as the puling babe, a grievous burden to themselves, and a disgusting spectacle to others, you would exclaim, as I have often done, 'Oh! the lamentable want of science that dictates the abuse of that noxious drug, calomel, in the Southern States!'

Gentlemen, it is a disgraceful reproach to the profession of medicine: it is quackery, — horrid, unwarranted, murderous quackery. What merit do gentlemen of the South flatter themselves they possess, by being able to salivate a patient? Cannot the veriest fool in Christendom salivate, — give calomel? But I will ask another question. *Who is it that can stop the career of mercury at will, after it has taken the reins in its own destructive and ungovernable hands?* He who, for an ordinary cause, resigns the fate of his patient to mercury, is a vile enemy to the sick; and, if he is tolerably popular, will, in one successful season, have paved the way for the business of life; for he has enough to do ever afterward to stop the mercurial breach of the constitutions of his dilapidated patients. He has thrown himself in fearful proximity to death, and has now to fight him at arm's length, as long as the patient maintains a miserable existence."

And this confessedly dangerous medicine is prescribed upon the most trifling occasion, even for infants, and for the most simple irregularities of digestion in adults. The susceptibility of certain individuals to its influence is very great; and a few grains may exercise upon such persons a powerful influence, which will cause for the time severe suffering, and be the means of permanent, irreparable injury. It is a well-known fact, that a spoonful of calomel is frequently given for a dose, even before the degree of susceptibility may have been ascertained; and, although with some no immediate perceptible injury is experienced, it is by no means certain that they will be freed from ultimate consequences of the most distressing character.

Professor Carlisle remarks, that "it seems passing strange that grave men should persist in giving large doses of calomel, and order these doses to be daily reiterated in chronic and debilitated cases. Men, starting into the exercise of the medical profession from a cloistered study of books, and from abstract speculations; men, wholly unaware of the fallibility of medical evidence, and unversed in the doubtful effects of medicines, may be themselves deluded, and delude others for a time: but, when experience has proved their errors, it would be magnanimous, and yet no more than just, to renounce both the opinion and the practice."

Calomel, however, is but one of many medicinal agents, to whose pernicious influence man sees fit to subject himself and others. *Opium* is another, well known and extensively employed, less directly destructive to organic substance than mercury, but acting with most deleterious energy upon the brain and nervous system; producing, in large doses, vertigo, convulsions, delirium, and death. In its different pharmaceutical forms, it is more generally used than any other medicine. In a pulverized state, it enters into most of the prescriptions of the physician;

and as laudanum, paregoric, &c. it is freely resorted to by men, women, and children. If it relieved pain and promoted rest, at all times and under all conditions, no reasonable objection could be urged against its general use, and it would indeed be a precious remedy; but this is far from being the case, for it is by no means constant in its operation as a sedative; and its primary action, if favorable, is certain to be followed by an action precisely the reverse. The nervous irritability and susceptibility to pain which may have been lessened for a short time by the first effect of the opiate, is greatly augmented when this immediate action subsides; and the existence of actual pain is less troublesome than the intolerable state of uneasiness which prevails during its secondary action. Opium-eaters cannot endure the agonizing mental and physical prostration which is consequent upon the brief excitement caused by the drug; and they strive, by repeated doses, to keep up the primary action, until the nervous system is deranged, the brain stupefied, the constitution ruined; and the miserable victim becomes a poor, worthless "mass of humanity," like the abject consumer of alcohol, — a curse to himself, an object of loathing and scorn to every man in his senses with whom he comes in contact. Hahnemann has clearly depicted the unhappy condition to which the immoderate coffee-drinker is ultimately reduced; but the effect of opium is to a far greater extent noxious, inasmuch as it is a far more powerful poison. All stimulating narcotics are possessed of the same pernicious property to a greater or less extent; and it is their unavoidably evil influence upon the human system which makes it madness for man to resort to them while in health, and folly to place any dependence upon them as curative agents.

As has been remarked with reference to calomel, there exist different degrees of susceptibility in individuals to the action of opium; and the amount of susceptibility cannot, of course, be determined until the drug has once been administered. Dr. Robert Christison, in his treatise on poisons, states that "very young children are often peculiarly sensible to the poisonous action of opium, so that it is scarcely possible to use the most insignificant doses with safety." That thousands of lives have been, by its various preparations, destroyed during infancy, there is not the least reason to doubt. That fatal results among adults, from its immediate influence, without reference to its prolonged, eventual action, have been numerous, — far more than the world has ever been made acquainted with, — is equally unquestionable. The queen of Charles II. died from the effects of opium administered by her physician during sleep, after her repeated refusals to take the prescribed dose, knowing from previous experience its injurious consequences upon herself. The particulars are recorded by Agnes Strickland, in the work entitled "Lives of the Queens of England." From the conspicuous position of this illustrious victim, attracting, as she did, the interest of a whole nation, the facts attending her decease could not be easily suppressed.

It will not be out of place to quote here certain observations relative to a few medicines in domestic use, by a writer in the "Medico-chirurgical Review," published in London. He writes as follows: "That which is commonly called a most innocent medicine may be the source of the utmost harm, if it be taken at an improper moment, or under unfavorable circumstances. Thus, *magnesia* has been productive of fatal consequences, from the ignorance with which it has been administered, or the perseverance in taking it, when it has failed in its expected influence. Masses unchanged have been found after death, closely collected together, or patches of the powder adhering with the utmost pertinacity to the intestines, because there had been none of the acid with which it should combine to be properly efficacious. Some very curious instances of this kind are upon record, and some of the cases have been, from the apparently suspicious circumstances, made subjects of legal investigation; for even death from arsenic has been supposed to have taken place, when examination has shown that magnesia has been its cause. *Manna,* simple as it is supposed to be, has been known to produce dyspepsia of the most obstinate character, and intestinal derangement of an alarming kind. *Castor oil*, one of the favorite popular remedies, frequently occasions not only excruciating pain, but causes the expulsion of that which lubricates and defends the lining membrane from injury ; and what has been supposed to be exfoliations have taken place, leaving behind a surface so irritable that months have elapsed before a normal state has prevailed. The neutral salts, those of *Epsom*, &c. are not to be trifled with. Dysentery and other diseases, and sometimes dropsy, supervene upon their injudicious use. *Gamboge*, which has been a fashionable medicine, is of all others the most uncertain and oftentimes the most pernicious: its influence is principally exerted upon the muscular fibre, and hence peristaltic action is increased. It has been known, from its stimulating power upon the muscles, to produce intus-susception. Even *senna*, which certainly comes nearer to a harmless domestic remedy than any other, is not so: it is not only a momentary cause of pain and inconvenience, but it leaves behind a very great tendency to those uncomfortable sensations, and more particularly if the liver have not been previously called into some slightly increased action, by which the bile is poured forth, and thus the general action of the intestinal canal been duly and properly augmented. These circumstances demand the very greatest attention and caution. Indeed, a catalogue of sorrows, occasioned by the indiscriminate and foolish use of purgatives, might be drawn up; but such is the headstrong tendency some have to doctor themselves, that it would be rather a curious than a useful task to undertake it."

The nature of individual medicines, their characteristics and specific action, need not here be detailed. It will suffice for the present purpose to state, in general terms, that emetics cause an entirely unnatural action throughout the alimentary system;—deranging every healthy process, inducing debility and sometimes death; while their operation is in no case, or to any extent whatever, *curative*, excepting in the single instance of the removal of foreign substances accidentally introduced into the stomach: that *purgatives*—their presumed beneficial agency, founded on a pathological doctrine, long since admitted to be erroneous—pass into and through an organ for which they are not intended, to exercise their irritating influence upon a delicate membrane, whose only safety is in their sudden repulsion, and eventually augmenting the very difficulty which they are employed to obviate: that *tonics* and *stimulants* increase any inflammatory tendency which may be present, and by their ultimate action aggravate the condition which they are intended to counteract: that *opiates* cause a moment's suspension of pain and restlessness, and hours of inquietude and agony: that *depletives*, in the form of bleeding, cupping, leeching, &c. abstract the vitality which the recuperative powers of nature require for her beneficent operation: in short, that the entire practice of drugging, in all its branches, acknowledged as of doubtful efficacy by numerous brave veterans who *have retired* from the field, disturbs, instead of assisting, that restorative process by which health is regained; and is, of all the influences to which men on this earth are subjected, the most pernicious and destructive.

It is believed that in no other country on the globe are drugs used to such a lamentable extent as in these United States; that nowhere else are the sad consequences, fairly attributable to their action, so perceptible. Now, this wide-spread evil has been promoted by medical men, who are presumed to be acquainted with the nature of the human organism, the laws of health, and the doctrine of diseases. And it is from the blind, empirical practice of such men, from their profuse and random-shot drugging, that *quackery* has originated; yielding dishonorable support to thousands of unprincipled persons, who dare, without proper preparation, to undertake the responsible ministration of the physician; approaching the "sacred precincts of a sick room" with impudent, arrogant assurance, or circulating their cruel deceptions through a venal press; reckless of all results but such as are of a pecuniary nature. Countless is the number of unsuspecting sufferers, who, tortured with pain and urgent for relief, are induced by the bold assertions of the quack to trust to their dangerous compounds, until their diseases have progressed beyond the reach of all human skill. Terrible will be the remorse of those who have thus trifled with human life, when the earth is to them but a remembrance.

CHAPTER X.

ON MENTAL CAUSES OF DISEASE.

The influence of the mind upon the body, the intimate connection of the moral with the physical, is a subject of the highest interest in relation to health, and should meet with special attention. Immaterial as the mental faculties are, they nevertheless are dependent upon the action of a material organ, — the brain: that organ is nourished by the same blood, warmed by the same life, governed by the same laws, as other portions of the frame. By want of exercise or by over-exertion, its vigor is impaired, its functions deranged, its destruction threatened; and as care must be exercised in the adaptation of external agencies to the requirements of the body, that health may be maintained and life enjoyed, so must it be with the mind, which has its seat in the brain. As emaciated muscle, softened bone, disorganized nerve, obliterated blood-vessels, may result from disuse, or injuries equal in extent from excessive use of the physical powers, so may the mental be disordered and destroyed by imperfect or extraordinary exercise.

An unhealthy condition of the mind from inaction is not unfrequently the unhappy lot of those whose calling comprehends a very limited range of objects, or who, provided with a sufficiency or superfluity of the earth's goods, suffer themselves to sink into a sort of mental lethargy, becoming resigned to an uninterrupted state of repose, and almost literally "thinking of nothing." Not caring to enter the wide field of literature; perceiving little worthy of attention, beyond their own worthless selves, in a world full of interest and excitement, they fall into inanity, but few degrees removed, seemingly, from the "beasts that perish." Those godlike faculties, qualified for engaging, with pure delight, in the loftiest contemplations and the most sublime investigations, with a boundless range for their exercise and expansion, capable of constant advancement in knowledge, step by step, for ever, are allowed by many to run almost to waste over a few mean, contracted notions, which blight the brain, and bring weariness and grief on the deathless spirit.

Intellectual food and exercise are as necessary for the health of the mind as material food and physical exercise are necessary for the health of the body. And as with the latter every part is to be exercised, in order that the whole may be invigorated, so, with the mind, each faculty should be in active operation. The resemblance may be continued; for as excessive bodily exertion tends to diminish instead of increasing vital energy, so extreme mental application, or violent exercise of the brain, debilitates the power of thought, and disposes to derangement. It is, of course, through its physical frame-work that the intellect is disordered by close application. The laws of the perishable material must be regarded, if we would properly realize the uses of our intellectual nature. The mind will not long act with vigor in this life, if the nervous system, with which it is most intimately connected, is in an unhealthy condition; and neither will the nervous system long continue in a normal state, while the mind is subjected to constant, unrelaxing exertion.

Powerful mental emotions prove always injurious, and sometimes instantly destructive to vital action. The physical condition is affected by the state of the mind, and on that condition depends the continuance of health and life. The nervous system is the most directly influenced by strong impressions upon the mind, and through this communication the impression is transmitted to all the physical functions. *How* the immaterial acts thus upon matter, how this wonderful union of soul and body exists, is an enigma that man cannot solve. He may ascertain the cause of an emotion; he may make himself familiar with its effects; he may, to a certain extent, neutralize its disturbing action upon the body, by remedies *dynamic* in their character, — but he can go no further. Mental suffering, from a distressing calamity, prevents the proper oxygenation of the blood, interrupting the circulation and disordering respiration. Alarm, on the approach of a pestilence, depresses the nervous energy, and debilitates the whole frame to such a degree that death's work is easily accomplished. Man knows this; but all inquiry into the nature of a connection so intimate is as unsatisfactory, as fruitless, as is the attempt to investigate the principle of life, to account for the sufferings of the pure and innocent, to penetrate any of the Almighty's deep mysteries.

The dependence of the body upon the mind, the close intimacy of the spiritual with the material, is in no instance more strikingly exhibited than when vehement passion takes possession of the soul. Falling heavily upon the brain, through that mysterious communication which God only understands, the dynamic, immaterial, yet overwhelming influence is transmitted through the nervous connection to the centre of circulation, and the heart *breaks*—literally. It is not always a metaphor, this sad "heart-breaking." There are on record instances of an actual rupture, from powerful emotion, of the muscular walls of this organ's cavities, producing instant death. When the emotion is not of that overpowering nature which kills at once, but is permanent and corroding, it makes itself seen and felt in perverted functions, disordered nerves, languid circulation, and deranged digestion.

Grief is a consuming passion, which, indulged in, gradually undermines the constitution, wearing out and wasting away life's energies. When the mind is dead to the blessed consolations of religion, there is no emotion so permanent and remediless, — none so generally injurious in its effects. Congestion and inflammation of the heart, insanity, apoplectic and epileptic fits, emaciation, impaired functions of every organ, result from grief. The best therapeutic measures are those belonging to homœopathy. The best hygienic influence is submission to the will of God.

Macbeth. Canst thou not minister to a mind diseased;
Pluck from the memory a rooted sorrow;
Raze out the written troubles of the brain;
And, with some sweet oblivious antidote,
Cleanse the foul bosom of that perilous stuff
Which weighs upon the heart?
Doctor. Therein the patient
Must minister to himself.

Anger, that terrible passion, which, when amounting to fury, transforms man into a demon, may, if violent and prolonged, cause hysteria, convulsions, hemorrhages, diseases of the liver, madness. In its lightest form, there is an accelerated flow of blood to the brain, and a disturbance of the nervous system. Many counteracting measures have been advised, such as the instant concentration of all the mental powers in forming a firm resolution for its immediate suppression; the stern compulsion of that "unruly member," the tongue, to silence; the careful avoidance of the rage-begetting monster, alcohol. But when the pitiably weak subject of an influence like anger, in its most fearful shape, urges the entire absence of self-control as a claim to indulgence, the most successful remedy would probably be the hydropathic application of the "douche;" for this overwhelmingly active refrigerant seldom fails to calm those enraged animals that cannot boast of reason.

Fear, *joy*, and the infernal passions of *envy* and *malice*, all act through the same communication noxiously upon the physical frame. It is not necessary to enter into an account of the peculiar effects of each. Dissimilar as the character of the above-named emotions are, their effects are not unlike. The same morbid phenomena, cerebral derangement in chief, with disturbed nutrition and cardiac affections brought on through the connection existing between the brain and other organs, are consequent upon intense excitement from all strong emotions, save that of *love*. No harm is produced upon body or mind by the cultivation of this divine attribute. We allude to the disinterested, holy love of the mother for her child; the creature for the Creator; the pure passion of one congenial spirit for another; the all-absorbing desire to add to the happiness of the loved object, unmixed with the base, calculating thought of self. There is no divinity in the form of this passion where selfishness dwells, and in that foul, earth-born sensuality, which the world often dignifies with the name of love. There is health, spiritual and physical, in the one; there is sickness, death, and "deep damnation" in the other. And when this cheering, celestial visitant enters the mind, it may be entertained and cherished without fear of its harming the body. It is not only innocuous, but it is a preservative of health; and the "blessed influence of that love which has followed the pardon of sin," has even *cured*, and will yet cure, many physical aliments that baffle human skill.

It will be understood that reference has been made, in the account of unhealthy influences from passion, to the consequences which arise from a high degree of mental excitement. The emotions, from which no human being is exempt, if not prolonged to the degree which enslaves and distorts and debases the mind, are not necessarily injurious to health. On the contrary, a quiet, well-regulated indulgence of the different emotions is believed by Combe and others to be salutary, and there is "a greater resistance to morbific impressions than when the functions are executed with a languid sameness."

To those who cannot, or who will not, comprehend the dynamic nature and operation of remedies, who persist in believing that there is no "more in heaven and earth than is dreamt of in *their* philosophy," the assertion that the "Stygian darkness" in which the *materialist* has long groped relative to the cure of mental distempers might be illuminated by the light which Hahnemann brought, will doubtless be read with incredulity, perhaps with contempt. Be it so. The homœopathic practitioner is too well shielded now to be vulnerable to the well-worn shafts of scorn and ridicule. He is not to be driven from his present position by such weapons. Homœopathy offers remedies directly curative for many of "those peculiar diseases of the nervous life and psychical stages of human maladies whose symptoms exhibit so much that is wonderful and mysterious, that the credulity of a dark age imputed their existence to demoniacal agency. These diseases bring us to the borders of a spiritual world, whose dark regions no beholder's eye has yet penetrated, and whose hieroglyphics no thoughtful mind has hitherto deciphered; and the therapeutics of the old school, in relation to the treatment of such affections, exhibit a struggle of the crudest materialism against the most obvious dynamical derangement."

We refrain from enlarging upon curative measures, since the subject is obviously inappropriate here; and conclude this chapter with the observation, that no high-minded, honorable physician will slight any suggestion made in good faith which may possibly tend to the alleviation of human suffering.

CHAPTER XI.

ON INVISIBLE INFLUENCES AFFECTING HEALTH.

Many agents which exert most powerful action on health and life are *imperceptible*. Surrounding and pervading all created things, they are silently operating throughout the universe, having no determinate shape nor definite proportions, forcing man to recognize their wonderful influence, and humiliating him with a sense of feebleness and dependence. Such are light, heat, air, electricity. And the principle of infection, — that strange, inscrutable agent, — whether generated from modifications of life-sustaining powers, or existing independently of them, is also imperceptible. It falls upon mankind with irresistible force, filling the world with lamentations of the living for the dead, and yet is known only by its terrible effects. If material, we are certain that the poison must be exceedingly minute; for it is not discernible by the aid of the highest magnifying power.

Through the agency of certain of the imperceptible influences, many inorganic substances send out emanations which are perceptible. Odoriferous particles, immeasurably small, occasion, through the olfactory sense, consequences often serious, and sometimes positively destructive. Headache, nausea, unconsciousness, are not unfrequently produced by the strong perfume of flowering plants. The daughter of Nicholas I. Count of Salin, expired immediately after inhaling the odor of violets. Henry VI. of Germany, and the wife of Henry IV. of France, were, as is stated in history, killed by perfumed articles of apparel. Many examples of this kind might be mentioned; but the establishment of the fact that invisible forces exert a wonderfully depressing action upon the vital powers need not depend upon isolated instances subject to doubt. All must be aware of the potency of these unseen influences. It is certain that they possess a strong innate power of action, capable of producing very decided effects; although, by reason of idiosyncrasy, they may operate more violently upon one person than another.

We have alluded to the consequences of malaria, in a previous chapter. Those consequences are sufficiently prominent. The sufferer feels them most sensibly, and the traveller cannot but perceive them instantly. Yet the cause, that mighty power which acts so powerfully, is without odor, taste, color, sound, volume, or dimension. It broods over the infected district perpetually, penetrating the organism of man and beast; and the highest mortal ingenuity is baffled in the detection of a single palpable atom of the poison. And so it is with the miasm of cholera, of small-pox, and other infections; each producing peculiar and distinct effects; each equally immeasurable, imponderable, imperceptible.

There are precautionary measures that may be adopted, to a certain extent, both by individuals and communities, — to which reference has been made in another place, — for partial resistance to agents so subtile and mysterious. It is not designed to treat here of those measures, but to endeavor to expose the unreasonableness of refusing to admit the efficient action upon the system, of any poisonous property, *because* it is not grossly material. When miasma can be reduced to masses of matter, and shovelled into druggists' shops; when electricity can be measured like Epsom salts, and caloric weighed like calomel, the time will have arrived when the ridicule which has been wasted upon "infinitesimal doses" of medicine will be more legitimately directed, and perhaps more influential, than it happens to prove at the present time.

There is a principle belonging to all those substances that disturb the vital force, which, according to Hahnemann, is latent in the crude drug. That principle is dynamic, as independent of substance as the soul is of the body. It can only act with unobstructed power, when the material which confines it is broken into fragments; and the development of that power is in proportion to the extent of separation of the particles. When these particles are separated, it is the released spirit of the drug, a peculiar, immaterial principle, which exercises upon the human system a specific influence, *sui generis;* each medicinal agent having a character differing from all others. This principle, concealed until disclosed by human labor, is the active power which corrects the abnormal condition of organic life, restoring health to the diseased frame. It is distinct from the grossness of matter, as distinct as is heat and light from earthly substance. The disengagement of electricity or caloric from bodies by friction is analogous to this development of medicinal virtue by trituration. There is nothing more incomprehensible, nothing more ridiculous, in one than in the other. No more do they form actual portions of the substance in which they are imbedded, than does the fragrance of the rose form the visible flower.

Now, certain diseases are known to be produced through agents not recognizable by our senses. Pestilential emanations have never been proved substantial; yet their energetic, penetrating power, the whole world is acquainted with. There must be a cause for effects so striking. That cause must be considered dynamic, in the absence of all proof that it is material. And, if the disturbance of vital action constituting disease is occasioned by a dynamic cause, why may not the removal of disease be effected through similar agencies? Strange, that, exposed as man continually is to deleterious influences from without, which he cannot but acknowledge act intensely, though undiscernible, he should find it so difficult to believe in the efficiency of minute agents, when applied internally and intimately to the sensible organs of life.

Should the animalcular theory ever be proved correct, and a material cause for epidemic diseases be established, the fact would still remain unaltered, that the most powerful action ever brought to bear upon human health is the result of forces excessively minute. Professor D'Amador asks, in the paper read before the scientific congress at Nismes, "What are relative greatness and smallness in the case of the seeds of vegetables, but a mere *lusus naturæ?* Who could believe that invisible seeds of plants are continually suspended in the atmosphere? that those of mosses, of fungi, of lichens, elude our eye, and float invisible in the circumambient air? Who could believe, if experience did not prove it to us every day, that within the case of a seed, which, from its minuteness, cannot be perceived by the microscope itself, there is contained the power that shall one day produce a vegetable? Who could believe, in fine, that in the embryo of the acorn there exists, in infinitely little, the largest tree of the forest, which only stands in need of development? According to Dodart, an elm can produce, in a single year,

529,000 seeds; Ray counted 32,000 on a stalk of tobacco. If all these seeds should come to perfection, it would only require a few generations, and a very small number of years, to cover the whole surface of the habitable globe with vegetables. If, then, atoms can produce an entire being, why should we tax them with impotence when the question is about merely modifying a being? If an atom gives life, is it more difficult to conceive that it may change the mode of being? When the *greater* exists and starts up before us in the processes of nature, why should the *less* be declared impossible?" And, in another part of the paper he adds, with reference to the agency of minute *medicinal* doses, "If the action of imperceptible agents is opposed to common sense, that is as much as to say that experience is opposed to it; but, as common sense and experience are not, and cannot be contradictory, if common sense refuses to believe in the action of imperceptible agents, common sense stands in need of a thorough reform, which experience will be able to effect. Science, which is nothing else than the reflection of experience, has, in this manner, reformed common sense several times. Common sense believed for centuries that the world was fixed, and astronomical science corrected common sense, and brought it to its own way of thinking. The virtue of vaccine was repugnant to common sense, at the period of its discovery; but now experience has so completely demonstrated it, that any one who doubted it would be held to be destitute of common sense.

"Why should we treat with contempt a system of therapeutics, which is but the application of one of our most certain maxims? To the diseased vital forces are opposed the forces of natural substances, but divested of all material covering: these forces will thus be brought face to face; they will act directly on each other, without any interposing agent; and hence will ensue rapid, certain, and agreeable cures. . . . . Observe, that the vital therapeutics of which I speak are to medicine what the study of electricity and the imponderables has been to chemistry; what the study of motive powers has been to mechanical art. . . . Far from overthrowing Hippocratism, or the true vitalism of Montpelier, our modern therapeutics confirm, complete, extend, and apply it, add what was wanting to it, and supply its deficiences. The divine old man bequeathed to us, so to speak, the code of medicine in which its great laws were laid down, its principles registered, its fundamental dogmas established: the work of ages is, and ever shall be, to deduce from these premises the most remote consequences; to bring all the great facts which subsequent discoveries may reveal and produce within the Hippocratic domain. Some of these discoveries have been already gathered in, and can never more be lost; others have been sown, and as yet exist but in the germ; but nought can blast this germ: on the contrary, it will grow, and the tree will yield its fruit to us and to all posterity."

CHAPTER XII.

ON HOMŒOPATHY.

Not many years since, a doctrine was broached in Saxony of a novel and extraordinary character. A long-sought desideratum in medical science was assumed to have been discovered; a brilliant light thrown upon the dark path of the groping, bewildered disciples of Æsculapius.

Samuel Hahnemann, a German chemist and physician, after years of laborious, untiring investigation, pursued with the earnest, all-absorbing interest characteristic of his countrymen, — after long-continued, closely studied experiments in developing and maturing into palpable form a conception elicited by accident, published, in 1811, a voluminous report of his labors. From this work we learn, that, twenty years previously, the author instituted certain experiments upon himself, while in health, with the view of ascertaining the true and positive action of cinchona (Peruvian bark) upon the system; being induced to this trial by the perplexing and contradictory statements published respecting the curative properties of this drug. He took several doses of a strong decoction of the bark in the morning, for many consecutive days, and uniformly experienced towards evening febrile symptoms, analogous in every particular to the fevers arising from marsh miasma. Astonished at the resemblance of the symptoms thus produced with those which this medicine is known to remove, he was led to suppose that the cure of disease consisted in this similarity of action. For the purpose of verifying his conjecture, he continued to experiment with other medicinal agents, long regarded as successful remedies in certain forms of disease. Ulcers in the throat, inflammatory glandular swellings, &c. were consequent upon the continued use of mercury. Cutaneous eruptions resulted from large doses of sulphur. And complaints of a similar character are known to be controlled by the judicious administration of those minerals. The three medicines referred to had acquired the reputation of "specifics." By what mode of action such a character had been established, under what law other than that of "*similia similibus curantur*" (like cures like) their "specificity" enrolled itself, it would puzzle pathologists to determine. After numerous trials, in all situations and circumstances, the consequences were the same. Different medicines produced distinct classes of symptoms, undeniable in existence, unchangeable in character. By comparing these results with subsequent experiments upon the sick, it was ascertained that convalescence became rapid and complete, whenever remedies were employed whose effects upon the healthy corresponded with the symptoms observable in disease; and, the closer this correspondence, the more immediate and decided was the recovery. Day after day, year after year, Hahnemann, with a few medical associates, pursued his investigations with uncommon perseverance and devotedness, anxiously watching the development of a great truth, seizing upon every circumstance favoring its elucidation, and sternly rejecting whatever would not bear thorough and searching criticism.

For more than two thousand years, therapeutics had been involved in doubt and darkness. Vague speculations, untenable hypothesis, influenced medical practice, for brief intervals, one theory being abandoned for another; while various conflicting methods of cure were at times distracting practitioners' minds, plunging them into a sea of empiricism, and bringing reproach and scorn upon the "art of healing." Cheering and most satisfactory had been modern progression in chemistry, medical botany, and operative surgery; but, in the absence of an immutable principle, a fixed foundation upon which to build, practical medicine had remained nearly stationary since the time of Hippocrates. The need of such a basis had constantly been felt and frequently expressed, and intimations of the existence of the homœopathic law had been given by Stahl, Bertholet, Paracelsus, Cardanus, Thomas Erasmus, and others. Haller proposed the administration of drugs to those in health as the only certain mode of accurately ascertaining their action. But no one before Hahnemann had undertaken systematically to *prove* the characteristic properties of medicinal agents upon the human economy, — to note the whole extent of their operation, — to register, with conscientious minuteness, every alteration effected by their influence. An intimate knowledge of the nature and operation of the weapons to be wielded by the medical practitioner had ever been most desirable, and that information was thus afforded. The want of facts as a groundwork for treatment had ever been deplored, and that want was thus supplied.

In the practical application of the homœopathic principle, a striking distinction prevails regarding the amount of medicine administered. In the crude state, as ordinarily given, neither vegetable nor mineral remedies were found to possess so much efficacy as when a division of their particles had been effected. The medicinal property appeared to be augmented in proportion as the substance approached the atomic condition. Certain materials which, placed in contact with the organism in a condensed form, are inert, become remarkably active when their particles are separated by friction. Moreover, an exceedingly feeble influence only is required to produce a very sensible impression upon a diseased portion of the body. An inflamed surface is affected by the slightest pressure; the faintest ray of light acts with painful power upon an inflamed eye; the stomach, in a state of inflammation, rejects the smallest quantity of nutriment. This excessive susceptibility is attendant upon inflammatory and other diseased action, and hence the *rationale* of "infinitesimal doses."

By a series of trials unparalleled in rigid scrutiny, Hahnemann claimed to have established, among others, the following propositions, viz.: —

That a group of morbid symptoms, from whatever cause arising, will be removed by that medicine which is capable of producing a similar class of symptoms.

That the curative property of medicines becomes, by undergoing trituration or succussion, greatly augmented; and that extremely minute doses are, in consequence, sufficient to counteract any diseased condition.

That the effect of medicinal substances is destroyed by combination, and their efficiency advantageously exercised only when administered singly.

Explanatory of the first proposition, it was remarked that remedies produced a train of symptoms which were manifestations of a medicinal disease similar to the natural one; and, as the existence in the system of two diseases resembling each other was impossible, the morbid must yield to the medicinal symptoms. The latter, dependent on the continued application of the remedy, will disappear when that remedy is discontinued, and the natural condition of the affected parts will consequently be restored. Or, again, the symptoms indicative of disease are but manifestations of the recuperative efforts of nature; and, as the medicinal agent operates in the same direction, it will aid the restorative process, and thus facilate recovery.

Respecting the second proposition, that the potency of medicines is greatly increased by a peculiar mode of operation, it is asserted that, in the crude state of a drug, its virtues, to a considerable extent, remain latent, and are only to be brought into full activity by a thorough breaking down of the enveloping material, and a complete separation of the molecules of matter. Only by the rapid motion of liquids, and the friction of solids, is the cohesion of particles to be destroyed. These two processes develop intense power, — as, for example, electricity,—which without their agency would have no existence; or, rather, would have existed in an inactive, dormant state. Whether the curative influence of medicine be disengaged by the minute division of particles, so that their mobility is increased, and placed more in affinity with the animal fibre on which they are to operate, or whether a new power is developed like electricity by friction, being transmitted by successive infection to inert substances with which it may be connected, diffusing itself to an almost unlimited extent, while preserving all its primitive qualities, are mere abstract questions, in the determination of which no point of practical importance is involved. Analogous facts of the disengagement of inherent force by friction, and of the influence upon corporeal substance even of impalpable, imponderable agents, are well known and universally acknowledged.

In relation to the propriety of rejecting medicinal compounds in favor of simple remedies, but few remarks are necessary. A heterogenous mixture of various substances, thrown into the system, conflicting with and counteracting each other, form a bewildering complication of drug-symptoms, that would blind the keenest sight, and embarrass the most discriminating judgment. A slight regard to the "improved" therapeutics and symptomatology would convince any one that a single uncombined remedy, judiciously administered, is sufficient, in any given case, to effect all that medicine can accomplish.

Under all methods of practice, cures have unquestionably been performed. The antipathic method, which is as old as Galen, and not by any means less faulty *because* more ancient, is directly the reverse of that inculcated by Hahnemann, and consists in the administration of remedies which, by their primary action, bring about a condition opposite to that which it is intended to remove. Combating isolated symptoms, and causing violent commotion in the organism, it, more frequently than otherwise, injures by repressing instead of assisting the re-action of nature. As a system, it is unphilosophical, incomplete, and pernicious. The same may be said of the revulsive method of the humoral pathologists, and the principle of counter-irritation, which, in nine cases out of ten, needlessly multiplies the sufferings of the unfortunate patient; burthening the exhausted frame with augmented incumbrance, and often irrecoverably disabling organs which were performing their functions in a healthy manner. Blistering, leeching, bleeding, cauterizing, homœopathy repudiates as in a majority of cases entirely useless, and in all cases decidedly barbarous.

In the investigation of diseases, for the purpose of curing by the above treatment, opinions as to the seat of the complaint are at once formed from a few prominent indications, and active measures are immediately put into requisition against a name. There *may* have been an error of judgment. It ought not to be termed invidiousness to assert that the practitioner is *sometimes* mistaken in his diagnosis. The means have been adopted, however, *secundem artem*, heroically depletive it may be, and the natural capacity of resistance to diseased action lost, perhaps for ever. Mistakes made in medical practice cannot *always* be remedied.

A painter, who had but little talent as an artist, embraced the profession of medicine. His friend inquired the reason for such a change. "In painting," replied he, "every fault is exposed to view; in medicine, they are all buried with the patient."

We transcribe from Rau: "As it would be unjust, on the one hand, to reproach a physician with the impossibility of establishing a correct diagnosis, when the means for so doing are wanting, so it would, on the other hand, be unpardonable to base a vigorous antipathic treatment upon a purely speculative view of disease. I will not here detail the dreadful errors which have been committed by theorists. Two things may occur, if the realization of a wrong theory in practice should lead to bad results. Either the physician is too vain to admit his error, and continues to heap sin upon sin; or else, aware of his mistake, he changes his view of the disease, and modifies the treatment accordingly. In this way he continues groping in the dark, and altering his plan of treatment from day to day. The pure effects of drugs, particularly those of the favourite compounds, being very little known, the most prominent symptoms of the remedies that are used in a case are frequently mistaken for new phenomena of the disease. This leads to new views about the character of the disease, and to a change of treatment. Our journals are filled with reports of cases by the most celebrated physicians, which betray the most woful vacillation between a pretended rational and symptomatic treatment. A gentleman living abroad, who is affected with a chronic malady, sent the writer a large bundle of prescriptions, together with the opinions of five celebrated physicians, who had leisurely examined his case. All those physicians differed in opinion, each taking a different view of the nature of the disease. All of them were mistaken."

The homœopathist is not content with a superficial examination of the sick. The whole assemblage of symptoms, all the accompaniments of whatever nature, the immediate and remote causes, the external circumstances which alter, and the moral impressions which influence to any extent, the morbid state under consideration, are to him all-important. He cares but little about nosology then. A complete portrait of the disease, so far as external manifestations can afford it, is what he purposes to obtain; and, this obtained, there is a remedy. That remedy is simple, safe, and certain. It acts by no revulsion, causes no commotion, disturbs in no degree either the mind or the body.

An excellent illustration of the homœopathic principle is given by Kaltenbrunner, in his description of microscopical discoveries in traumatic inflammation. He is explaining the natural process through which the morbid inflammation is dissipated by the development of a state perfectly similar to it, which is termed the curative inflammation. "After a wound has been received," he remarks, "there commences an accelerated motion and a turgescence of the blood in the vessels surrounding it. From this point, those alterations extend to a greater or less distance. In some of the smaller blood vessels nearest to the wound, the motion of the blood is thrown into disorder, some canals become entirely emptied, in some it accumulates in irregular masses; while, in others again, it diffuses itself into the parenchyma, forming reddish islands of blood, at the same time the perenchyma beginning to smell. Driven with accelerated motion, masses of the globules of the blood, here and there, rush by starts from their canals, and pour themselves into the parenchyma of the inflamed part. Here they lie as bright red spots or islands of different sizes. Soon the whole wound is surrounded by these islands, and the intervening parenchyma becomes highly turgid. This process, which appears at first at the circumference of the inflammation, by degrees involves also the centre, and resembles the morbid inflammation completely; and it is by its means that the alterations produced by the latter are gradually extinguished."

A distinguishing feature in the homœopathic system is the importance allowed to mental affections in the selection of remedies. Although, by reason of the acknowledged intimate connection of mind and body, the pathology of the old school recognizes the necessity of attending, in some measure, to the condition of the former, yet in no mode of practice heretofore adopted have specific medicinal influences been directed to the state of the mind exclusively. No *materia medica*, except that of Hahnemann, prominently distinguishes moral derangements, or treats of immediate means for their removal. His experiments have established the important fact, that medicines, operating upon the human structure, not only alter its vital functions in a peculiar manner, but exercise a characteristic action upon the spiritual existence, — the mind and disposition. According to Mayerhofer, this truth can be made use of as an available point in therapeutics; and upon this field of pharmacodynamic psychology, the founder of homœopathy appeared not simply as a reformer, but as a creator of a new world, hitherto shut out from pharmaceutic investigation.

Another marked distinction in Hahnemann's doctrine is his theory of chronic diseases. He asserts that the multifarious affections of the skin from which mankind, the youthful portion especially, suffer, are but indications of an internal virus, termed *psora*, which has been transmitted from parent to child for ages; that inveterate chronic ailments are, in most cases, owing to the sudden repulsion, by local applications, of the secondary vicarious symptoms of this virus, externally manifested. Many proofs are adduced in corroboration of this statement; and there are few practitioners who have not witnessed the occurrence of serious internal maladies after the suppression of a cutaneous eruption, and a singular inability in patients of resisting attacks of an acute disease arising subsequently to the forced removal of such an eruption. Hahnemann adds that the appearance of the psoric disease is especially favored by an irritable, vehement temper; by the exhaustion consequent upon unusual physical exertion; by improper medical treatment, excesses at table, and dissolute habits. Owing to its peculiar nature, the psoric virus may remain latent under favorable circumstances. In this case, the patient appears to enjoy good health, until some untoward cause rouses the internal disease, and causes it to break out. Neither the relatives nor the patient, nor the physician himself, can comprehend how it is possible that his health should have declined in this way so suddenly. The diseases which then make their appearance, even after a trivial accident, as fractures, &c. cannot be traced to any cause: they return in spite of a first successful treatment, and of the strictest diet; they increase each time they reappear in the system, especially in the fall or spring; and finally settle down in the form of a lingering malady, which cannot be treated according to the rules of the allœopathic practice, without exposing the patient to the danger of having a more severe disease substituted in the place of his former ailment. There are innumerable causes which may rouse the internal psora, and cause it to develop its manifold germs: the evil effects of those causes often bear no sort of apparent relation to them, which renders it difficult to consider them the true exciting causes of the secondary psoric disease, the often fearful character of which ought, on the contrary, to be explained by the existence of a deep-seated, latent disturbance, which has broken out on this occasion, and is the common mother of all such chronic secondary affections.

The doctrine that chronic diseases are caused by a virus infecting the system, and also, not unfrequently, by over-doses of medicine taken for the purpose of curing them, receives an unexpected and very decisive confirmation from the fact, that, under hydropathic treatment, favorable changes in the sick are preceded by the appearance of pustules, ulcers, &c. upon the skin, and always by excessive perspiration, having the distinct odor of certain medicinal substances which have been taken at some previous period, often long distant. Happily, however, the neutralization of the virus referred to may be obtained by a much less severe and painful method, viz. by the cautious and judicious employment of remedies answering homœopathically to the morbid effects of this virus, which, if not allowed to settle in the system, may, without difficulty, be completely eradicated.

Thirty-nine years ago, the "Organon" was published. Since that time, the method of practice therein taught has extended throughout Europe and America. Public attention was first earnestly attracted by its astonishing success in the treatment of Asiatic cholera in Hungary. Hospitals were from that period founded; professorships were granted; and its extension has since been unprecedented in rapidity. Among its present adherents are nineteen professors in European colleges, twenty-three state counsellors, seventeen medical counsellors, and fifty-four eminent army surgeons, besides an innumerable body of well-educated private practitioners; and it has never been more flourishing than during the present year, notwithstanding the assertions to the contrary of its opponents. Of four professors in different European universities who have publicly made a trial of homœopathy, but one has declared against it: that gentleman is Prof. Andral, of Paris. The three of the four who declared in its favor, and now openly recommend its practice, are Prof. D'Amador, of the University of Montpelier; Prof. J. W. Arnold, of the University of Zurich; and Prof. Henderson, of the University of Edinburgh. The published, unquestionably veracious statistics from medical institutions in Vienna, Berlin, Leipsic, London, Paris, Naples, and other cities, in most instances under the immediate supervision of civil directors, prove incontestably, by the small proportion of deaths and "dismissed incurables" under homœopathic treatment compared with the allœopathic practice, the very great superiority of the former over the latter. Such advocates as Quin, Jahr, Henderson, Arnold, Jourdan, Horatiis, Stapf, and Cramer, all of whom hold some of the highest medical stations in Europe, are not to be lightly esteemed. No "humbug" ever enlisted minds of such an order. The hackneyed, oft-refuted arguments of the wilfully blind affect not, with a feather's weight, the ponderous mass of evidence already existing, and constantly accumulating, in the progress of homœopathic practice. Were medicine a perfect science, instead of being lamentably and confessedly inadequate, no opposition to innovation could be too combined and inflexible. But, when the oldest and most distinguished men in the profession have distinctly and publicly affirmed that medical records are little else than collections of fluctuating opinions, of versatile, ephemeral views, changeable as the fashions, abounding with conjectures, and conclusions drawn from premises "baseless as the fabric of a vision," — a disclination to deviate from the old graveyard-path is indeed surprising.

That the above remarks may not be deemed illiberal and unauthorized, we quote the opinion of Dr. Forbes, the former editor of the "British and

Foreign Medical Review," a gentleman of acknowledged talent and extensive professional reputation. He thus writes concerning allœopathic practice, which, while deploring its deficiencies, he strangely pursued. With this quotation, our fragmentary essay will terminate: —

"The comparative powerlessness and positive uncertainty of medicine is exhibited in a striking light, when we come to trace the history and fortunes of particular remedies and modes of treatment, and observe the notions of practitioners, at different times, respecting their positive or relative value. What difference of opinion! what an array of alleged facts directly at variance with each other! what contradictions! what opposite results of a like experience! what glorification and degradation of the same remedy! what confidence now, what despair anon, in encountering the same disease with the very same weapons! what horror and intolerance at one time, of the very opinions and practices which, previously and subsequently, are cherished and admired!

"To be satisfied on this point, we need only refer to the history of any one or two of our principal diseases or principal remedies; as, for instance, antimony in fever, blood-letting in pneumonia. Each of these remedies has been at different times regarded as almost specific in the cure of the two diseases, while at other times they have been rejected as useless or injurious. What seemed once so unquestionably, so demonstrably true, as that venesection was indispensable for the cure of pneumonia ? and what is the conclusion now deducible from the clinical researches of Louis and others ? Is it not that patients recover as well, or nearly as well, without it ? What are the opinions and the practices of the surgeons of the present day, and the indubitable facts brought to light during the last thirty years, with regard to mercury ? . Are they not, that it is unnecessary (generally speaking) to the cure of those cases for which it was once thought specific, and that it is often most injurious, in place of being beneficial ? The medical god, mercury, however, seems as unwilling to be balked of his dues as the mythological. If he has lost his former domain, he has gained another, that of inflammation ; and many of our best practitioners might possibly be startled and shocked at the supposition that their successors should renounce allegiance to him in the latter domain, as they themselves had done in the former. And yet such a result is more than probable, seeing that there exists not a shadow of more positive proof (if so much) of the efficacy of the medicine in the latter than in the former case.

" The same truth, as to the uncertainty of practical medicine generally, and the utter insufficiency of the ordinary evidence to establish the efficacy of many of our remedies, as was stated above, has been almost always attained to by philosophical physicians of experience in the course of long practice, and has resulted generally in a mild, tentative, or expectant mode of practice in their old age, whatever may have been the vigorous or heroic doings of their youth."

Taking into consideration that the foregoing remarks are from the most eminent medical reviewer — the highest allœopathic authority — in England, the most ardent reformer of medicine could not expect, and would not demand, a more candid admission.

THE END.

www.ingramcontent.com/pod-product-compliance
Lightning Source LLC
LaVergne TN
LVHW011236110826
845150LV00006B/1650

* 9 7 8 1 4 2 5 5 1 4 4 2 6 *